THE
HAND OWNER'S
MANUAL

A Hand Surgeon's Thirty-Year Collection

of Important Information and Fascinating Facts

by

Roy A. Meals, M.D.

"The Hand Owner's Manual," by Roy A. Meals, M.D. ISBN 978-1-60264-266-9.

Published 2008 by Virtualbookworm.com Publishing Inc., P.O. Box 9949, College Station, TX 77842, US. ©2008, Roy A. Meals, M.D. All rights reserved. No part of this publication may be reproduced, stored in a retrieval system, or transmitted in any form or by any means, electronic, mechanical, recording or otherwise, without the prior written permission of Roy A. Meals, M.D.

Manufactured in the United States of America.

To Susan

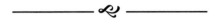

*whose love, support, sense of good taste, and gentle critique
greatly enrich my writing and my life*

TABLE OF CONTENTS

INTRODUCTION

T HIRTY-FIVE THOUSAND TEACHERS HAVE HELPED ME
prepare the material for *The Hand Owner's Manual*.
These are my patients. They range in age from newborns
to centenarians and span the social spectrum from homeless to
celebrity. For work and recreation they use their hands in
ordinary and amazing ways. Pain, stiffness, numbness, and
limited use are often the causes of their concern, and it is my
privilege to help relieve these problems. I find it particularly
challenging and rewarding work for two reasons. Our hands profoundly affect how we physically interact with the world, and
they also affect our mental state. They are visible to all and reflect our ages, habits, and personalities. On a daily basis we take
their function and appearance for granted, but even the smallest
paper cut or blemish can make us acutely aware of these compact, complex, durable marvels. Aristotle described the human
hand as the "tool of tools." I am honored to be its repairman.

As with any subject scrutinized over time, patterns emerge
from apparent chaos. For me, a professional lifetime of reading,
attending and presenting papers at meetings, dissecting in the
laboratory, and especially talking to patients have revealed
nuances about the ways hands work, fail, and heal. These ways

would be invisible on short or casual observation. This makes my work fun, always interesting; for, in fact, I have 35,000 teachers, and new ones push me forward every week.

In 1994 I began writing a semiannual newsletter for my teacher-patients. I have two goals for each issue. First, I want to share my experience and excitement about how hands work and how readers can prevent injury and, when necessary, nurture healing. Second, I want to celebrate the hand's pervasive influence on the entire human story. So I cover topics as diverse as our base 10 numbering system, sign language, and hands in movies. It pleases me to hear that the newsletters are anticipated, read, discussed, and passed on.

The Hand Owner's Manual draws from the newsletter and has identical goals: share and celebrate. Thanks to all 35,000 of my teacher-patients who have knowingly and unknowingly contributed. Thanks also to my son, Clifton, who has among his many talents a gift for drawing. His illustrations are scattered throughout the book and contribute to its light-hearted tone, which helps make learning fun. If Aristotle knew of *The Hand Owner's Manual,* surely he would join the celebration.

CHAPTER

1

HANDS

Through the Ages

L ONG AGO PRIMITIVE SHARKS HAD RIDGES RUNNING down their sides from gill to tail. Later, muscles grew into the folds, and eventually the central portion of each ridge receded while the ends enlarged to form fins both fore and aft. All was well.

Then one day several hundred million years ago, a fish was swimming blissfully in a shallow pool. The tide went out and much to the fish's surprise, she could use her five-rayed fins to move around a bit on the rocky bottom. The tide came in and she swam away, never to give this event another thought. The world, however, was forever changed.

For many generations thereafter, that fish's offspring went back to the pool and progressively got better at moving across the rocky surfaces on their fins. Some even started squirming short distances overland from pool to pool. They developed pockets in their throats that could absorb oxygen directly from the air, which was far more efficient than deriving oxygen from moving water through their gills. Not only was breathing more efficient on terra firma, but also plant food was abundant and there were no predators. The fish slowly developed stronger skeletons, waterproof skin, and longer fins. They now walked and hopped and only returned to the water when they laid eggs. Amphibians were born. Birds and reptiles were next; the sequence is under some dispute, but those fins were now assuming various shapes to facilitate flying, running, and even fighting. For now there were competitors.

Then mammals came along with warm blood, hair rather than feathers or scales, and the ability to nurse their young. The earliest mammals were tiny and entirely intimidated by the dinosaurs. They wisely kept out of sight; but when those terrible lizards bit the dust, mammals came out of their crevices. Some went to the mountains, others to the plains, some to the trees, others underground. The ones who adapted most efficiently to their new environments survived and thrived.

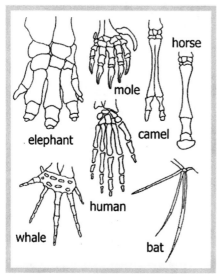

Mammals assumed many sizes, shapes, hair colors, and habits. Those pectoral fins from their fish ancestors became amazingly diverse and particularly suited for special purposes on land. Various habitats favored different adaptations. Long fingers in some instances favored reaching the best berries and eggs. Sharp claws in other instances could shred bark or competitors. For elephants, their noses evolved into their grasping appendages, capable of uprooting trees and picking up peanuts. Elephants, therefore, benefited more from broad, thick weight-bearing platforms for hands and feet than they would from five dexterous digits. Other large animals found no use for five digits and efficiently adapted to their environmental niches with fewer. The rhinoceros has three digits, the camel two, and the horse only one, best for running, which horses do on their fingernails--well, hoofs.

Some mammals found life on the land too dangerous or competitive and went underground. Moles, with strong tunneling tools for upper limbs, are particularly well adapted for this life.

2

An extra bone, which at first glance looks like a sixth finger, widens the hand.

A few mammals found a special niche by taking to the air. Bats still have five digits, but they are as thin as the elephants' are thick. The thumb retains a claw useful for crawling, and the index and middle fingers are fused together to form the primary strut. Thin webs of skin stretch from fingertip to fingertip to provide tools for flight.

Other groups of mammals decided that life in the ocean was not all that bad and rejoined their fish ancestors. Sea otters continued with paws and claws, while whales and seals developed flippers for maximally efficient swimming and for chasing their fish relatives.

Then there are human hands—not really that good for anything. We can't bear hundreds of pounds of pressure on them while we pull down trees with our noses. We can't walk on them for weeks across hot sand or run a mile in two minutes on our fingernails. Nor can we flap our elbows and fly, swim the oceans for our entire lives, or burrow across the neighbor's lawn. Ah, but here is the beauty of the human hand—not terribly good at any one thing, but pretty good at a lot of things. We can bear some weight on them and we can swim a little. If we need to run we can use our feet. This frees our hands to use tools rather than to be tools. Need to dig? Pick up a shovel. Need to cut? Grab scissors. Need to fly? Build an airplane or reserve a ticket online. Even fly away for a fishing vacation. Just respect the fins on those scaly creatures you catch and know that you share some ancestors.

WHEN ANCESTRAL MAN FIRST STOOD UP

When ancestral man first stood up, he could see farther across the savanna and identify dangers from a distance. That was a good thing. But raising his center of gravity and balancing on just two limbs reduced his stability. That was a bad thing, and it has only gotten worse.

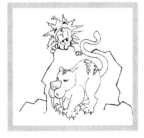

Uneven pavement, parking lot barriers, snowboards, mountain bikes, icy patches, unstable ladders, and crumpled throw rugs have all increased the chances of us falling back onto all four limbs. When that happens, we instinctively throw our hands out to break the fall. Often, we not only break the fall, we also break our wrists. Orthopedists call such an injury FOOSH— fall on outstretched hand. When toddlers begin to topple over, they just bend their knees and take a cushioned landing on their bottoms. Somehow by about age two, we lose this wrist-saving mechanism and FOOSH injuries then pursue us for the rest of our lives. Young children, older children, young adults, and older adults all have their own characteristic type of wrist fractures. So the treatments vary.

The bones in young children are very resilient and capable of some bending. If the bone does finally bend enough to break, it behaves like a green tree branch, not breaking cleanly but cracking and buckling with the two fragments maintaining some attachment to one another--hence their name, greenstick fractures. Kids have an incredible capacity to heal. Usually three weeks in a cast from palm to forearm is all that is needed to get them back on the monkey bars.

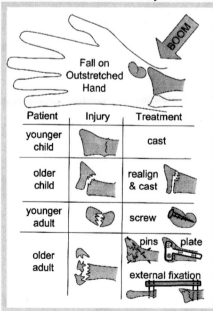

After age eight or so, our bones are not so rubbery, and the forces of FOOSHs have to be absorbed elsewhere. In older children the break typically occurs through a specialized region near the end of the bone. This is the region where the bone normally gains length during skeletal growth. This area is weaker than the bone itself. Bam!-- and the end of the bone slips partway off the shaft. The orthopedist can generally manipulate the fragments into satisfactory alignment. Thereafter the resiliency of youth again prevails, and skateboarding resumes after three to four weeks in a cast.

For the rest of us, it is not so simple. The weak link in the system for young adults is not the forearm itself, but a weirdly shaped wrist bone called the scaphoid. That means boat in Latin, but only one with a vivid imagination could name it so. Think of a bloated, warped inflatable raft. With a FOOSH, the boat cracks in two, and because the bone has a quirky blood supply, healing is slow. This means a minimum of three to four months in a cast, which would be irksome to a skier but financially devastating to a new dentist. Therefore, scaphoid fractures are often stabilized internally with a stainless steel screw. The patient thereby avoids a cast.

As we get on in years, we tend to lose our memory, our keen eyesight, our balance, and calcium from our bones. All of these factors contribute to wrist fractures, which now revert into the major forearm bone the same as when we were children, but now requiring twice as long in a cast to heal—at least six weeks. In that length of time, the wrist and fingers can irreversibly stiffen, muscles weaken, and the bone, now brittle and possibly shattered like broken glass, can settle into deformed and unsettling positions.

Various surgical treatments are available to foil this outcome. If the bone fragments are not shattered and just moderately unstable, steel pins may suffice. With multiple fracture fragments and more instability, plates and screws often help. Sometimes the bone is so shattered that trying to fix the fragments to each other would be like trying to nail a custard pie to the wall. In this instance, application of an external frame can temporarily bypass the crumpled area. (Think of it as a scaffolding that holds a bridge up while a supporting column is under repair.) This external frame attaches to the skeleton on both sides of the fracture by steel pins that protrude through the skin. Yes, it sounds gruesome, but it solves a difficult problem and it is a guaranteed conversation starter. Think of it as the cost of having a better view across the savanna.

CAST TREATMENT FOR FRACTURES

Ancient Egyptian embalmers preserved mummies by wrapping the dead in linen roller bandages. Five-thousand-year-old papyruses record that physicians also applied linen roller bandages to stabilize fractures and restore skeletal stability in the living.

Twenty-five hundred years later, Hippocrates described the then well-established art. "It should be done . . . quickly by dispatching the work; without pain, by being readily done; with ease, by being prepared for everything; and with elegance, so that it may be agreeable to the sight."

The bandage developed strength according to the number of fabric layers, especially if each layer was thoroughly rubbed with a mixture of lard, wax, rosin, or pitch. Some surgeons preferred a paste of flour and egg white. Based on local availability, strips of wood, sheet lead, hard leather, bark, or bamboo provided further rigidity. These methods did not change until the 19th century. Then three things happened. The urban population of Europe grew quickly. Surgeons were in short supply. The Napoleonic Wars inflicted many casualties. Doctors needed simpler means of fracture care. (Consider it a health care crisis.) Military surgeons learned that they could leave rigid dressings in place for weeks or even months, and fracture healing would be complete at time of bandage removal. Laundry starch and cardboard strips became the preferred materials. These dressings were slow to dry, but after several days, patients could be ambulatory and out of the hospital (cost savings).

Surgeons sought stiffening materials that would dry faster. Plaster of paris showed promise. At first, they placed the injured arm or leg in a shallow trough and poured it full of liquid plaster. This promptly hardened to immobilize the fracture and make a "cast" of the mold. The treatment was quick but left the patient with an extremely heavy and awkward bandage.

In 1851, a Dutch military surgeon came up with the idea of rubbing dry plaster of paris powder into coarsely woven fabric strips. He then moistened each strip just before rolling it on. To this day, wet fabric strips saturated with plaster of paris are rolled on over a thin layer of cotton padding. The padding prevents pressure sores from forming against the unyielding plaster. Unfortunately history does not record the name of the first patient to have his cast signed.

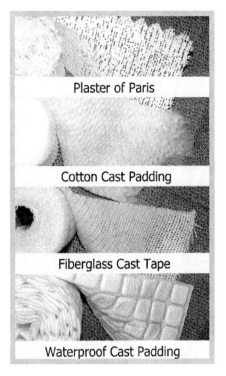

Plaster of Paris

Cotton Cast Padding

Fiberglass Cast Tape

Waterproof Cast Padding

Two modern-day embellishments of the age-old roller bandage are noteworthy. In some instances fiberglass has replaced plaster of paris. It comes in bright colors. Like plaster of paris, it also is activated by water and hardens quickly, but only fiberglass is waterproof. The cotton lining, however, is not, and remains soggy for days after an ill-advised swim or shower. A new, nonporous, cast-lining material looks somewhat like Bubble Wrap™ and lets water inside the cast quickly drain away. It is expensive, so some of the cost savings of ambulatory fracture care also drain away. The new cast liner does, however, allow patients the opportunity of wetting their skin and thereby smelling less like mummies.

Do you need to dress up a cast or splint to match your image for a wedding, anniversary, or other high-style event? Find a sock that complements your outfit. Cut the toe out of it. Several inches back from the end, cut a side hole for your thumb. Pull the sock over your hand and bandage like a fingerless glove. Party on, knowing that Hippocrates would have found it agreeable to the sight.

GOING DIGITAL

Not long after our ancient ancestors stood up and quit using their hands for locomotion, they could gather bird eggs, clams, berries, and other delectables. This posed several problems, however, if they took the bounty back to the communal cave. Who gets how many? How many times since the last full moon has Lazybones foraged for the group? Ancestral man needed a calculator, and the one closest at hand was, well, the hand. It is not surprising that "digit" means a finger or toe as well as a number. Primitive accountants used all the fingers and toes to get to 20, then they put a notch or score on a stick and started over. A score of 100-pound weights makes a ton, 20 pennyweights make an ounce, and an English pound used to equal 20 shillings. With

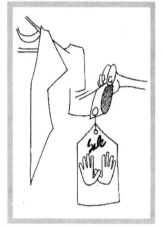

the advent of shoes, toes were excused from calculations, and our base-10 numbering system ensued.

In some tribal languages the same word means both "hand" and "five." Likewise, the Roman numeral **V** represents the open hand with digits spread widely, and **X** comes from both hands opened fully with thumbs crossed. Ancient merchants used different finger positions on the left hand to represent all the numbers from 1-99. The right hand recorded the hundreds. The Roman poet Juvenal wrote, "Happy is he who has postponed the hour of his death so long and finally numbers his years upon his right hand."

Several centuries later, Bede, an English monk and historian, extended the system of finger reckoning. The left hand demonstrated one- and two-digit numbers. The right thumb and index represented the hundreds and the right middle, ring, and small fingers represented the thousands. Left hand placement over the breast, thigh, navel, or hip with the palm facing either inward or outward signified the 10,000s, and identical placements of the right hand took care of the 100,000s. Clasping the hands overhead with fingers interlocked denoted a million. Lottery winners still sometimes demonstrate this same notation.

Early writings imply that finger reckoning was extended to perform addition and multiplication. Cicero, for instance, noted that fingers were necessary to determine the difference between simple and compound interest. He did not record whether all these manual gyrations led to forms of overuse syndrome among moneylenders.

Here's a simple system for multiplying numbers up to 10x10 using the original digital calculator. Let's multiply 9x7. First subtract 5 from the 9 and turn down four fingers on one hand. Then subtract 5 from the 7 and turn down two fingers on the other hand. Add the turned down fingers (4+2=**6**) and multiply the turned up fingers (1x3=**3**). Voilà, **63**. For the algebra nuts, it's ab=[(a-5)+(b-5)]10+(10-a)(10-b). Actually, it might be easier just to learn the multiplication tables. Either way, keeping your mind agile may allow you to eventually count your age on your right hand.

RULERS ON HAND

At some point in time, ancestral man began cutting captured game into steaks rather than roasting the entire carcass on a spit. Soon members of the tribe began wanting their share grilled to order but refused to let the cook test the doneness with a knife, which let the tasty juices escape. Chefs learned to poke the steaks with their finger to determine how well it 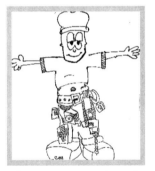 was cooked. Meat gets firmer as it cooks, so assessing its squishiness against a readily available norm (your hand) still works. Gently pinch the thinnest part of the web between your thumb and index finger—that soft feel equates to rare. Move a half inch closer to your wrist and pinch again—that is medium rare. Then on the palm side, poke the firm muscles at your thumb's base—that is well done.

When early humans could count, they could also start to measure more than just money and age, but that required rulers. Imagine ancient man being caught at a primitive fabric or office supply store, lumberyard, or horse auction without a measuring stick. His sense of doom must have been the same as ours, weighing the inconvenience of finding a ruler versus "eyeballing" the measurement and then getting home to find that the new acquisition didn't fit. Before you find yourself in that age-old position again, take a minute to calibrate your built-in rulers.

Originally the distances for an inch, foot, and yard were derived from readily available standards. The span of your arms is almost identical to your height. Therefore, the distance from your nose to your fingertip is half your height. That's a yard if you are six feet tall. If you are not exactly six feet tall, you can still closely approximate a yard by turning your head toward your hand if you are taller and away from your hand if you are shorter. Calibrate this distance with a yardstick. Then you can easily measure off yards of rope, fabric, jungle vine, or any other flexible material, although unknowing bystanders may think you are just smelling it.

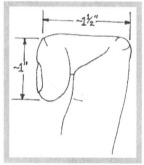

The span of your stretched out hand from tip of small finger to tip of thumb is another measurement, seven to ten inches depending on the size of your hand. Measure it. Then you can just move your hand across an object inchworm fashion and multiply the number of hand spans by the width of your span.

For smaller measurements, your flexed index finger works well. From fingertip to your first joint is close to an inch, and from the first to second joint is about an inch and a half.

And of course, when measuring horses, it is the width of your palm (four inches) repeated from the horse's hoof to shoulder. A Shetland pony stands about 10 hands high and a Clydesdale up to 17 hands.

THE HAND IN SPIRITUAL LIFE

Throughout human existence, the hand has had a pervasive role in religion. Many of the early civilizations overlapped in time and geographical location and influenced one another. Therefore, saying which concept or practice came from which religion is difficult, but here are some interesting connections between the human hand and spiritual life through the ages.

The hand is one of the well-known symbols of the Hindu deity Shiva, who transforms one life into the next and whose hand is the token of life and might. Various gods of life and fertility in Babylonia, Assyria, and Phoenicia are depicted with an uplifted hand, and clay tablets from this time in Mesopotamia designate "prayers of the lifting of the hand." The uplifted hand continues into modern times as a gesture of blessing and confirmation, and over the ages it has found its way into various secular swearing-in ceremonies.

During the time of Egyptian Pharaoh Akhenaten, about 1300 BC, stone carvers depicted the sun god as a disk from which rays stream, each ending with a human hand. These solar fingers caress and support the bodies and crowns of Akhenaten and his

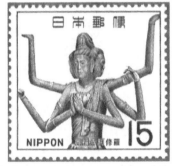

queen. Other ancient gods had multiple hands to represent their invincible strength and power. Aizen Myo-o, the Japanese god of love, had six. Agri, a chief god mentioned in the Hindu Vedas, had seven. Guanyin, the Buddhist goddess of mercy, performed her compassionate acts with as many as 1000 hands.

Beyond the number of hands, their postures provide rich symbolism for the world's religions. Some Jewish rabbis make a two-handed gesture during their benedictory blessing. Their hands are raised, palms turned outward and fingers extended. The tips of the thumbs touch as do the tips of the index fingers, while

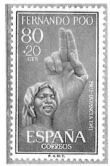

the middle and ring fingers form a V as the middle finger is kept close to the index finger and the ring finger is kept close to the small finger. The "live long and prosper" salute of the Vulcans on *Star Trek* is a modern-day, one-handed version of the same gesture.

In Christianity, followers began making the sign of the cross in the second century AD. In Eastern Orthodox Churches, the thumb, index, and middle fingers are brought to a point symbolizing the trinity of the Father, Son, and Holy Spirit, while the ring and small fingers are folded into the palm and represent the human and divine natures of Jesus. In Churches of the West, the fingers are held open and represent the five wounds of Christ. In Christianity as well as in nearly all of the world's religions, one-handed gestures are made with the right hand, which is considered holy, while the left hand is the sign of the devil.

Buddhism ascribes elaborate symbolism to the hands. The fingers represent the natural elements beginning with the thumb for water and the other fingers in sequence for space, earth, fire, and air. Contact between certain fingers signifies a merging of

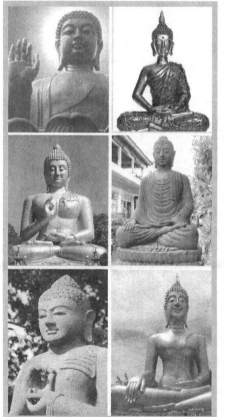

different elements and reflects the belief that all matter consists of the basic elements in varying proportions. The right hand symbolizes a man's capacity for physical work. The left hand symbolizes a woman's quality of wisdom.

From the fifth century onward, artists have sculpted Buddha's image to represent his sacred nature. With a deep understanding of Buddhist symbolism, a skilled artist can infuse the sculpture with a wealth of subtle meanings. Hand gestures, called *mudras*, are among the most symbolic and denote momentous events in the Buddha's life, which became key principles of Buddhism.

The right hand raised with palm turned outward signifies protection. Both hands in the lap with right hand over left represent disciplining the mind through meditation with the left hand's wisdom supporting the right hand's capacity for work. The raised right hand with the tips of index finger and thumb touching symbolizes education. The use of both hands to make thumb-index circles signifies the attainment of knowledge and the obligation to share it with others. The mudra with the palm turned outward represents generosity. With the palm turned downward and the fingers touching the ground, this mudra symbolizes the power of concentration to overcome worldly temptations.

Among the most ancient of gestures used by mortals is one person touching another to transmit power, endow a mission, or provide a blessing. In the Old Testament for instance, Israel blesses his grandsons, Ephraim and Manasseh, by placing his hands on their heads, and later Moses lays his hands on Joshua and commissions him to lead the Israelites. The New Testament tells that Jesus took the children in his arms, placed his hands on their heads, and blessed them. For centuries, Jewish teachers have "graduated" their students by laying on hands, giving them the authority to teach independently. Catholic bishops confirm and consecrate priests by touching their exposed heads. The same gesture found its way into baptisms and confessions. Followers of Eastern Orthodox Christianity kiss their priest's hand as part of a ritualized gesture of greeting and blessing.

The priest-physicians in Egypt and Babylonia may have been the first to use touch for the sake of healing. Both Old and New Testaments refer to laying on of hands as a means of healing. For instance, in Luke 4, "After the sun had set, people with all kinds of diseases were brought to Jesus. He put his hands on each one of them and healed them." In the 1600s and 1700s, lines of kings in both England and France practiced the royal touch, healing with their hands. Cervical lymph node tuberculosis was common and became known as the king's evil, because these royals were called upon to heal it by the laying on of hands. Several kings also handed out coins during the healing ritual, and there remains some uncertainty as to how many of the subjects came to acquire health versus wealth.

Other impious distortions include calling the fingers the ten commandments. Shakespeare's Duchess of Gloucester, quarreling with Queen Margaret, expounds, "Could I come near your beauty with my nails, I'd set my ten commandments in your face." In Longfellow's *Spanish Student*, the gypsy thief commands his men, "As soon as you see the planets (candles) out, in with you, and be busy with the ten commandments. . . ."

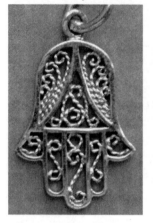

A belief, also ancient in origin, is that a person could suffer misfortune if looked upon with envy, be it for wealth, beauty, health, or offspring. Many cultures call this look the evil eye, although malice is not necessarily intended. Particularly in the Middle East, many people wear amulets known as *hamsa* hands or *hamesh* hands to ward off this form of bad luck. Predating both Judaism and Islam, the amulet usually is two-thumbed and symmetrical and represents the hand of a goddess that could stop the evil eye. *Hamsa* (Arabic) and *hamesh* (Hebrew) mean "five" and refer to the fingers. In Islam the fingers represent the religion's five tenets, which are profession of faith, prayer, pilgrimage, fasting, and charity.

Hand symbolism even extends beyond death. Symbolic carvings often embellish gravestones, particularly those from Victorian times. Hands pointing upward are said to point the pathway to heaven, clasped hands denote either farewell or a marriage bond, praying hands are asking for eternal life, and blessing hands are gesturing those left behind, who, as you will see, may need to ante up some prayers for the recently departed.

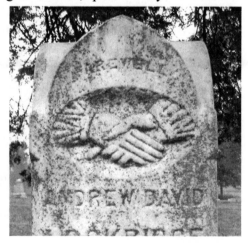

FIERY HAND PRINTS

If you find yourself in Rome with time on your hands, check out the Museum of Purgatory and the implications of having fire on your hands. As Catholics know, purgatory is the state between heaven and hell where spirits must make amends for their sins before passing through the pearly gates. Friends and relatives praying for the recently deceased can hasten this transition. Apparently dwellers in purgatory have at times dramatically reminded the living to pray more intensely and frequently on their behalf.

Would receipt of a fiery print of the deceased's hand motivate prayer? The Museum of Purgatory thinks so and reflects on this form of instant messaging. The story starts in 1731 when the recently deceased and stranded soul of Friar Panzini scorched his hand's image onto a wooden table at his former monastery and clutched at the sleeve of a nun's tunic, leaving burn marks.

The one-room museum adjacent to the Church of the Sacred Heart houses a collection of such artifacts gathered over 100 years ago during a priest's travels throughout Europe. The current curator recognizes that the collection attracts as many skeptics and "paranormalists" as it does believers but feels that a visit at least opens a discussion about Catholic ideas. See you there? Museo del Purgatorio, Parrocchia S. Cuore, Lungotevere Prati 12, 00193 Roma.

HANDS INVADE ENGLISH

When early humans started making sounds to represent numbers, they also needed sounds to express basic concepts such as man, woman, sun, eat, and go. In fact, these words, along with hand, have existed in English as far back as scholars can trace. English now has approximately 600,000 words and continues to borrow freely from other languages to sustain itself as the most expressive and nuanced language on earth. It is easy to understand how the concept of hand expanded into words such as handy and handle; and handsome originally meant easy to handle. Is it easy to handle a handicap? A betting game, "hand in cap," required the players to hold their money in a hat and then withdraw their hand, with or without their money, depending on the announced odds. Later, a superior racehorse carried extra weight, a handicap, to even the contest. From there, handicap also took on the meaning of encumbrance or disability.

The concept of hand is more widespread in English than you may imagine, partially because it manifests itself in disguised forms. Take manifest, for instance. Hand in Latin is *manus,* and when the Romans invaded England way back when, they brought a wealth of words all related to hand: manual, manage, manacle, manuscript, mandate, manipulate, manufacture, manner, manicure. Edmund means prosperity-protector; the mund comes from--you guessed it--*manus.* A further disguise hides *manus* inside words, for instance, emancipate and amanuensis, which means "one who takes dictation." Today, a secretary could fill a pamphlet with such *manus*-derived words that marched into English directly from Latin. Maintain maneuvered itself indirectly into English from Latin by way of French.

So, what about the French? They invaded England too. What did they leave? Well, they left pamphlets and manure—at least the words. Pamphlet comes from Old French *paume-feuillet,* a leaf of paper held in the hand. Manure is a contraction of the Old French, *manouvrer,* meaning manual work, which tilling and amending the soil certainly was. Increased fertility resulted from this legerdemain (*léger de main* - "quick of hand"). Another word for magic is prestidigitation, which was coined by a Frenchman in 1830 and is roughly based on Latin *praestigiator* ("juggler") and digitus ("finger") and influenced by the Italian presto ("quick").

The Greeks never invaded England, but their language did. *Cheir* is Greek for hand, leading to chiropractor, chirography (hand writing), and chiromancy (palmistry). *Ergon* is Greek for work. *Cheir* and *ergon* added together, *cheirurgos,* means working with the hand. The Romans messed with the spelling and turned it into *chirurgia.* In Old French that is *cirurgie,* and in Middle English, *surgerie.* So hand surgery is literally and accurately hands working with hands!

Our hands have come a long way from finny fish to a sentence such as this. *The handsome surgeon emancipated*

Edmund from his handicap and managed to manipulate the ensuing manuscript into a pamphlet and a manual—both feats of legerdemain, pure prestidigitation.

The true magic, of course, is how our hands develop from a microscopic fertilized egg in the first place.

CHAPTER

2

HANDS

Through Life

I STUCK MYSELF WITH A HYPODERMIC NEEDLE THE OTHER day. Intentionally. The first time in over 25 years of doctoring. More surprising, a six-year-old patient told me to do it, so I had to.

The boy, whom I'll call Tyler, came to the office with his father and had a large ganglion cyst on the back of his wrist—bigger than a jellybean. I told Tyler and his father all about ganglions and their treatment and my advice to drain it with a needle. Tyler didn't say anything when I mentioned "needle," but his eyes and body language told me that he wasn't liking the idea. His father in a loving way told him he needed to be brave, that some things just have to be endured. I added the standard (and true), "It's a very little needle. You'll hardly feel it." I sprayed a cold liquid first on my hand, then on his father's hand, and then on Tyler's to demonstrate its pre-needle numbing effect.

Even so, his facial expression told me that he wasn't going for it. Struggling to control his tears, he asked to see the needle. I showed it to him. Then with astounding wisdom he blurted, "If it doesn't hurt, stick yourself with it." I took a deep breath and thought, *wow, how am I going to make lemonade out of lemons?*

"If I stick myself, then will you go through with it too?" With his assurance that he would, I sprayed my wrist cold, tried to disguise my hesitancy, and stuck myself while he watched intently for any sign of a flinch. "Not fun, but not horrible," I related calmly.

Tyler climbed into the security of his father's lap and embracing arms. He buried his face and put his hand on the table. I drained his ganglion without hearing a whimper. Tyler and I got Band-Aids. We all left the room with a heightened multi-generational respect, courtesy of our amazing hands.

For me, the amazement begins with understanding the hand's fetal development and continues with its growth through adolescence and then with its century-long durability. In this chapter, I will share these fascinations and discuss several common disorders that predictably occur at various points along the road called life.

AN AMAZING JOURNEY

I remember as a child planting a few radish seeds in a foot-square plot that I had roughly cultivated. I was flabbergasted three days later to see that those hard little grains had transformed themselves into two-leafed solar collectors punching out of the soil. None of the radishes reached maturity because I was regularly pulling them out to assuage my excitement and curiosity. I still consider a sprouting seed to be an amazing display of life's renewal; but as complex and incompletely understood as it is, a germinating radish pales in comparison to the complexity of our own beginnings.

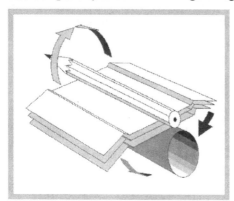

Consider this analogy. Imagine laying three hand-kerchiefs over an empty paper towel roll and then laying a pencil on top. Now pinch up the handkerchiefs a little along each side of the pencil to make ridges. Now make the ridges higher and fold them to-ward each other to cover the pencil. At the same time, wrap the free edges of the handkerchiefs around the paper towel roll. Understand that this same pattern of ridging and wrapping happened to all of us.

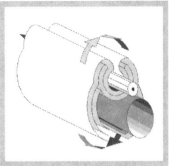

Every animal starts its journey into life as a single fertilized egg cell, which divides multiple times to become a microscopic ball of seething potential. For species that have spinal cords, the sphere flattens and elongates into a shield-shaped mass of cells after a few days. Then the folding occurs. It is the same for all vertebrates from sharks and frogs to birds and humans. The pencil represents our spinal cord. The paper towel tube represents the intestinal tract. The handkerchief represents three layers of different types of cells that will become everything from skin and bone to liver and lung.

At this point the embryo is still so small that it could sit comfortably on the head of a pin, but the cellular activity and differentiation that is occurring is miraculous. At one end of the spinal cord a significant enlargement occurs: the brain. By day 22 of development a nest of muscle cells begins to contract rhythmically. This is the heart. Along the way our gills and tail disappear, and by day 26, the part that makes humans unique, the hand, begins to develop.

It starts as a tiny bud from the border of this folded shield, which by now has assumed the characteristic fetal position but still measures barely an eighth of an inch in length. Each day the limb bud grows longer and then the end flattens. By day 36 of development, the paddle-like end of the limb has five scallops on its border. It also has five ridges that are oriented like a sunburst and that will form the bones in the palm and digits.

Over the next 10 days the fingers become fully shaped, and the webs between them recede. The thumb moves to its characteristic position and the arm bends for the first time at the elbow. Other joints quickly follow and come under the influence of early muscle activity and the first electrical impulses from the brain.

By seven weeks limb development is complete. The fetus, now three-fourths of an inch long, spends the next 30-some weeks just growing larger and stronger and adding some refinements. Skin creases in the palm appear at eight weeks, fingernails at 10 weeks, which is when fingerprints, which I will discuss later, begin forming. By 20 weeks the mother feels movements and the baby may begin passing time by sucking its thumb. At birth, only the nervous system is incomplete and will remain so for another two years.

Genes, specifically DNA, store the information needed for this miraculous transformation. Biologists are beginning to understand some of the DNA's protein messengers that leave sharks with gills and fins and advance us to lungs and hands. Some of the messages are extremely subtle and affect one cell but not adjacent ones. The exact influence is unknown. Why, for instance, do fingernails form on one side of our fingers but not on the other? How does a unique fingerprint end up on every finger of every individual?

Things can go wrong if a mutation alters the DNA data bank. Then the developing embryo gets an erroneous message. Other times normal DNA sends a perfectly fine protein message, but it may be blocked or garbled because of other chemicals swirling nearby. For instance, high maternal alcohol ingestion can cause certain limb abnormalities. Of course, the worst time to cloud the message is during those critical first seven weeks of development, some of which pass before the mother even knows she is pregnant.

Most times, we just do not know what went wrong when a child is born with a missing hand or extra or webbed fingers. I don't despair at the rare misinterpretation of the plans. Rather I marvel at the usual perfect execution of them, especially when considering our exposure to a myriad of trace chemicals in our industrialized and sometimes polluted environment. Imagine an entire suburb of new homes or a parking lot full of new cars being as glitch free as the usual new baby who began just nine months ago as a single, microscopic cell. Consider further that the human is far more complex and durable. It truly is an amazing journey and we all end up pretty much alike, but not exactly.

RIDGES, CREASES, AND WRINKLES

Upon scrutiny, individual variation is greatest on our fingertips, and interest in fingerprints is as old as human civilization. Prehistoric cave dwellers in Nova Scotia painted pictures of hands that included ridge patterns on the palms and fingers. Ancient Babylonians and Chinese businessmen closed transactions by pressing their fingerprints onto clay tablets and seals. Seven hundred years ago, a government official in Persia noted the uniqueness of every human fingerprint. A cousin of Charles Darwin was the first to study fingerprints systematically, providing a classification system for different patterns in the late 1800s. He also documented their individuality and consistency through life. Prisons and police departments gradually became interested, and the FBI started its repository in 1924. Its current biometric database contains over 55 million sets of fingerprints Computers have greatly reduced the tedium of storing and comparing these intriguing signatures.

The combination of genetics and environment makes each fingertip unique. Ten weeks after fertilization, the fetus, less than an inch long, has completely formed fingers. The shape of each tiny fingertip is genetically controlled, so its shape, be it bulgy, oval, or flat, is similar to that of the parents. Each fingertip's form will determine the general pattern, an arch, loop, or whorl of the yet-to-be developed prints. Over the next 12 weeks ridges appear in the digital skin. Fetal growth causes the ridges to spread apart; then additional ridges form and fill the spaces. Subtle differences in pressure and tension cause unique patterns in each ridge set. Who knows, are the differences related to fetal position, maternal sit-ups, tight clothes, laughing? Identical twins inherit identically shaped fingertips and have similar ridge patterns. Each tip, however, experiences its own microenvironment and forms unique, distinguishing details.

What purpose does this specialized finger skin serve? Much the way tire tread helps a car grip the road, friction ridges assist with secure manipulation of objects. Fingertips have an advantage over tires because each friction ridge comes with its own moisturizing system, sweat glands, to enhance traction.

This moisture may also enhance clairvoyance. Palm readers fathom your personal uniqueness by studying your hand's creases and high areas. They interpret your life line, heart line, sun line, fate line, and head line along with the intervening mounds, which are attributed to various planets and their astrological implications. Being a skeptic, I suspect that while holding your hand they are also assessing your age, body language, clothes, speech, nails, calluses, paper cuts, rings, and car keys. Even behind a perfect poker face, moisture from your friction ridges reveals excitement or nervousness, which palmists can incorporate into their interpretation of your future. I wonder how they would do if I stuck my hand through a hole in the wall and kept quiet. They probably could not tell my fortune, but they could pretty accurately guess my age because those clues are readily apparent.

Babies' hands are of course small, but their fat layer conceals joints and veins and gives them their characteristic chubby appearance. As we gain in years, we lose elastic fibers. We sag and wrinkle, and hand skin is no exception. It also becomes thinner, which reveals the contour of underlying joints and the network of bluish veins. Much of this is inevitable, but regular use of sunblock slows the process and prevents at least some local discolorations. Later in the book I will discuss cosmetic hand surgery, but for now, I want to answer a question I am asked all the time.

IS KNUCKLE CRACKING DANGEROUS?

Do you know how a carbonated drink fizzes when you first open it? Carbon dioxide dissolved in the liquid forms bubbles when you pop the top and release the pressure. The same phenomenon can happen in our joints because nitrogen gas that we inhale disperses in all our tissues. By stretching a joint and reducing its pressure, a bubble of nitrogen briefly forms with a popping noise. Is knuckle cracking dangerous? Obnoxious, maybe, but not dangerous. This bubble-forming phenomenon is perfectly harmless to the joint.

How about finger sucking? Bones respond to the forces that are applied to them and slowly alter their shape and density to resist those forces. Based on this principle, braces align teeth by slowly altering their position within the remodeling bone. Teeth will also move against the pressure of a sucked finger, although not where an orthodontist would want them to go. Logically, but less well known, while the finger is pushing on the teeth, the teeth are pushing equally hard on the finger. Finger deformities ensue and may require surgery to bring the digital pacifier back into satisfactory alignment for keyboard activities and appearance. A child has to suck intensely for 10-12 years to deform a finger, so it is not a common occurrence, but an awareness of the phenomenon is a great way to introduce bone as a remarkable, responsive, living tissue.

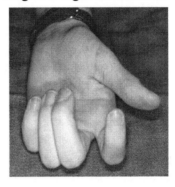

HOW BONES GROW AND HOW KIDS CAN STOP THEM

Have you wondered about how we get from roughly 20 inches long at birth to three or four times that tall in adult life? The simple answer is that our bones get longer. How they get longer though is fascinating.

Most of our bones attach together end to end. These connecting points, of course, are joints where cartilage caps the specially shaped bone ends. The cartilage, slick and springy, lets our joints glide smoothly. If a bone grew longer from its end like a bamboo shoot gets taller, there could be no cartilage caps. Even infants would be creaky, rubbing raw bone ends together. Instead, there are chemical factories a short distance back from the bone ends that produce a mix of protein and calcium crystals. These areas are called growth plates. They deposit new bone and in so doing, push the cartilage caps ahead. The growth plates automatically disappear when we are teenagers, and when they do, we are finished growing. Until then, these high-energy bone factories are fragile. If a growth plate is injured and disappears

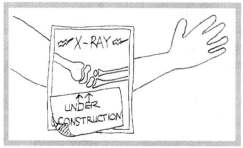

prematurely, the bone is short. This causes a limp if it occurs near the knee or an unnatural arm angulation if it occurs near the elbow. Either is a prelude to arthritis and lifelong problems.

Sudden damage to the bone, such as fracture or infection, is an obvious way to jeopardize the growth plate's health. A child may subtly cause damage by trying to be a little adult on the baseball diamond or in the gymnasium.

Little league elbow is a catchall term for a collection of ligament and growth plate injuries, all bad, in the growing arm. Kids see their favorite major league pitchers hurling fast balls over 90 miles per hour and want to mimic them. Think about it, though. The only way the ball can get going that fast is for the hand to push it. This whipping motion is not natural or healthy. Pros tolerate it because they are paid well. Kids do not know what is happening to them, especially if an overzealous coach or parent is hollering, "No pain, no gain, Champ."

The same thing can happen to the wrists of pre-teen girls performing gymnastics. Our bodies are designed neither to hurl baseballs nor to walk on our hands, much less to do handsprings off the vault at a dead run. Such repeated forceful impacts can damage one of the growth plates in the forearm. First the wrist becomes sore. Repeated impact injuries cause the bone to stop growing.

For a young Olympic hopeful with a sore elbow or wrist, rest is best. Once the pain goes away, the doctor will likely allow a moderate level of the inciting activity, as long as the area remains painless. The emphasis should be on technique, not repetition. Prevention, of course, is best. With this in mind, Little League Baseball instituted new pitching rules beginning in 2007. Players younger than 11 years old can only throw 75 pitches in a game before a reliever is required, and anyone who throws 21 pitches has to give the arm the next day off to recover. Sliders and curve balls contort the arm even more than fast balls and require extra practice to perfect them. So save breaking pitches for high school after the growth plates in the arm have taken the bones to their natural adult length.

With additional years, individual variations continue to manifest themselves. Some are related to our genetic make-up, some to our activities, and some for no clear reason. Certain conditions, however, typically affect individuals of one age or another. For instance, babies are unlikely to have heart attacks, and grandmothers do not typically get appendicitis. Hands have age-specific problems as well. Here are several common hand maladies that seem to appear sequentially as we move through life.

BIBLE BUMPS

People are justifiably alarmed when lumps suddenly appear on their wrists. The lump's owner may become distraught if a relative or friend offers to bash the lump with a heavy book. Besides, librarians take a dim view of this Victorian-era treatment. Is there a better approach?

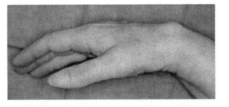

Many of these wrist growths are ganglions. Ganglion means "knot," and these fluid-filled lumps are the most common tumor of the hand

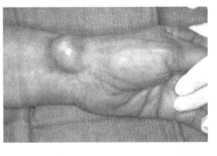

and wrist. For unknown reasons, ganglions appear in people 20-40 years old with far greater frequency than in those who are younger or older.

Ganglions most often occur on the back of the wrist in line with the thumb and index finger. Depending on the tautness of the enclosed fluid, the ganglion may feel either soft or hard. Often it is painless, but sometimes it presses on a nerve and causes pain, particularly when the wrist is in an extreme position for push-ups or downward-facing dogs in yoga.

The next most common location for a ganglion is on the palm side of the wrist at the thumb's base. If it wraps around the artery where one normally feels the pulse at the wrist, the "knot" may seem to be throbbing. The ganglion may then be mistaken for a problem with the artery.

Ganglions can also occur at the base of the fingers where they join the palm. Here they never get much larger than a BB gun pellet and are therefore not visible. They cause pain, however, with forceful gripping against hard objects such as a gearshift knob or briefcase handle.

Without a clearly understood cause, ganglions arise from the flexible ligaments that surround our joints and tendons. The thick fluid in ganglions resembles corn syrup in color and consistency and is the same chemical composition as the fluid that lubricates our joints and tendons. Because they are filled with fluid, ganglions can wax and wane in size, and sometimes patients accurately recognize that the lump appeared overnight.

Folk remedies include giving the bump a resounding thump with a heavy book. This bursts the cyst wall and allows the body to reabsorb the enclosed fluid. In a medical office, the less dramatic but equivalent treatment is drainage with a needle. Withdrawing clear, thick fluid confirms the diagnosis.

Depending on the activity of the area producing the fluid, the needle treatment is curative about half the time. Other conditions in the hand and wrist may mimic a ganglion, so doctors do not recommend indiscriminately bashing bumps with books for either diagnosis or treatment. Ganglions that recur after needle drainage and lumps from other causes may require surgical removal.

CARPAL TUNNEL SYNDROME

While young adults are prone to ganglions, older adults are prone to carpal tunnel syndrome. This condition was hot during the 1990s. Personal computers became commonplace. With them came the possibility of prolonged keyboarding and mousing without the need for any rest. No slapping the carriage return, inserting new pieces of paper, or manually correcting typos. Every ache from the elbow to fingertips quickly was tagged as the dreaded carpal tunnel syndrome. At the same time, a new technology came along for carpal tunnel release surgery—the endoscope. Doctors had a new tool to wave at the epidemic.

So where do we stand now? First of all, carpal tunnel syndrome existed long before keyboards and computer mice did. The condition is a nerve compression at the wrist. This nerve supplies sensation to the thumb, index and middle fingers, and part 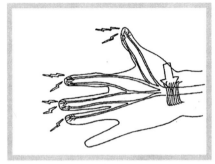 of the ring finger. It also provides control for the muscles at the thumb's base. When compressed, this nerve "goes to sleep" and causes tingling in the fingertips. With prolonged pressure on the nerve, the muscles around the thumb waste away, and numbness in the fingertips makes buttoning and other fine manipulations difficult.

Faulty sleep posture often contributes to carpal tunnel syndrome. The nerve gets pinched if the wrist is held in 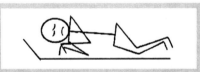 an extended (arched back) position or especially in a flexed position for a prolonged period. This impairs the blood supply to the nerve, and symptoms ensue. Repeated pressure leads to constant symptoms. So curling up to sleep with wrists tucked beneath your chin may feel secure, but it risks nerve damage. Wearing night braces that protect the wrists from extreme positions is often curative for early and mild symptoms. Likewise, avoid tucking your hands under your body, because this habit also cuts off the circulation to the nerve.

In many instances, carpal tunnel syndrome just happens—totally unrelated to keyboard or other repetitive activity. Should numbness and tingling persist despite taking the above measures, a precise medical diagnosis is the next step.

Severe and long-standing cases of carpal tunnel syndrome require surgery to relieve pressure on the nerve. Carpal tunnel surgery is usually performed on an outpatient basis with local anesthesia and possibly some light sedation. The surgery is generally quite effective in relieving symptoms, but the operation got somewhat of a bad name during the '90s because some people had the surgery and did not get better. Two factors contributed. First, not every ache in the forearms and hands is carpal tunnel syndrome. So if someone was misdiagnosed, treatment for one condition would be unlikely to relieve the other condition. Second, people were having the surgery and then returning to abusive levels of repetitive activity.

Finally, endoscopic carpal tunnel release has not proven to be all that great. As large numbers of patients have been carefully studied, the purported advantages of the high-tech procedure—diminished surgical site tenderness and less time away from work—melted away. Additionally, the endoscopic procedure proved to be more costly and time consuming; and even in experienced hands, it risks injury to incompletely seen structures. So the conventional, open procedure is generally considered the best.

Now with voice-activated computers coming along, archeologists in the *next* millennium may find computer keyboards adjacent to carpal tunnel endoscopes in their excavation trenches.

LET THE SURFER BEWARE

An interesting article appeared several years ago in the highly reputable *Journal of Bone and Joint Surgery*. It was titled, "Evaluating the Source and Content of Orthopedic Information on the Internet—The Case of Carpal Tunnel Syndrome. "

The authors queried five popular search engines to locate websites offering information on carpal tunnel syndrome. They took the top (first) 50 sites from each search. After eliminating duplicates, they evaluated the 175 unique websites for authorship and content and scored the informational value of each website on a scale of 0 to 100.

Nearly two thirds of the sites were businesses, one half of them selling products for the evaluation or treatment of carpal tunnel syndrome. Physicians and academic organizations authored less than one fourth of the sites, and an equal fraction offered unconventional or misleading information. The average informational value of the websites was 28 out of a possible 100 points.

The authors concluded that the Internet is presently a poor source of accurate information on this common medical condition. By extrapolation, other medical conditions are probably equally mishandled.

Undoubtedly the quality of medical information on the Internet will change as more academic organizations only publish information that has undergone a peer-review process to ensure thoroughness and accuracy. In the future, there may be something akin to the Good Housekeeping Seal of Approval for websites with valuable content. Several websites presently worthy of review are emedicine.com, webmd.com, aaos.org, and hand-surg.org. Under any circumstance, it would be wise to tell your doctor what you have learned (or think you have learned) about your condition both from your neighbor and from the Internet.

THE CELTIC CURSE

"Patrick, what's wrong? Your eye's all red."

"Mornin'. Yeah, I keep poking it when I wash my face. See, I can't straighten out my fingers anymore. And this palm thickening started a couple of years ago. Now it keeps my fingers bent. It's gotten so 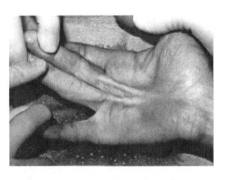 I can't even put my hand in my pocket, clap, or play the piano—almost anything I do with my hand flat, even shaking hands."

"I noticed. I thought you'd been giving me some secret handshake. But now I see you've got the Celtic Curse."

"What are you talking about?"

"I'll tell you while we work. You inherited that from your Celtic ancestors. Wales, Scotland, Ireland, England. All that was Celtic turf."

"OK, Wise One, so my mother's Irish, but my father's German. How d'you explain that?"

"The Celts got around—especially to Scandinavia, other parts of northern Europe, even Spain. They spread their genes pretty widely, and you don't need much Celtic blood to get it."

"How do you know so much about it? D'you read palms on the side?"

"My father has it. I took him to his doctor last week. It's called Dupuytren's contracture."

"Doo poo what?"

"Doo-peh-tren—it's the name of a French surgeon from about 1830. He was one of the first to operate on it."

"Surgery! Oh man, I don't want to get cut on."

"Well, like the doctor told Dad, it's not dangerous. It never kills anybody. It's not cancer. But it can be annoying when you can't get your hand flat. And since Dupuytren's time, every option has been tried—braces, massage, electricity, you name it."

"What are these cords? Are they the tendons? I need my tendons. I need my tend. . . ."

"Calm down. No, the cords develop from a thin layer of fibrous tissue just under the palm skin and sometimes on the arch of your foot. It's called fascia. It steadies the skin against the bones so we can hold onto things without the skin slipping around. It serves the same purpose as a pad under a throw rug. For some unknown reason, this fascia slowly thickens and shortens in some people with Northern European ancestry."

"Well, Mum doesn't have it. At least I don't think so."

"Doc said it's more common in men than in women and that it can skip a generation, so you may be right."

"I wonder about Patrick Junior. I'm German-Irish and Carla's Swedish."

"Yes, but Pat's just a teenager. The doctor said it's rare to see or feel anything before middle age. Even then, the thickening and shortening can be unpredictable—maybe not changing for years, then curling a finger in over six months."

"That's sure my story. Three months ago I could reach an octave. . . Mmmaybe I should… What'd the doctor tell your dad about surgery?"

"It's done as outpatient surgery. They sedate you a little and numb your arm, no need to be put clear under. Dad can start using his fingers after a few days, do some stretching exercises for about six weeks, then back to golf."

"There must be options. I know always to ask about options."

"Some surgeons try weakening and stretching the cord in the office by perforating the cord with a hypodermic needle, and there is an enzyme injection aimed at dissolving the cord that is showing promise in experimental trials. But for the pattern and degree of Dad's involvement, Doc said that surgery was best."

"Is he gonna do it? I've never heard of the Celtic Curse."

"It's more common that you think. About one in 20 Americans has at least a touch of it, and the older you get, the more likely it's there. Yes, Dad's surgery's tomorrow. And that reminds me. I' m going to take him, so I'll be in around noon. Don't forget to wear your green. Saint Patty's Day Parade starts at three!"

"TRIGGER FINGER? I'VE NEVER TOUCHED A GUN."

Trigger finger is the easier-to-say name for one of the most common things that goes wrong in the hand. Stenosing tenosynovitis is the clinical name. Whatever it is called, the affected finger sticks in a bent position and then it may hurt when the finger snaps straight.

When it is stuck, the finger vaguely resembles a gun's trigger, hence the name. So, trigger finger is completely unrelated to gun ownership. Infants get it in their thumbs. Then it pretty well skips over older children and young adults, but middle-aged and older people can get it, most commonly in the middle and ring fingers and the thumb. Adults who have one trigger finger eventually may have others.

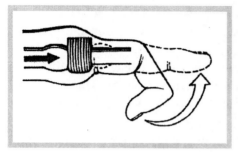

What's the cause? The main muscles responsible for making a fist are located in the forearm and connect to the bones in the fingers by tendons, which are tough, cord-like structures about the diameter of a thin wood pencil. As the tendons pass from the palm into the fingers, they enter narrow tunnels that hold them against the bones. Normally the tendons glide smoothly in and out of the tunnels as we contract and relax our muscles to open and close our fists. Occasionally and for no obvious reason, a tendon develops a thickened area that doesn't slide easily into the tunnel. Then it takes extra force to snap the tendon's thickened portion in and out of the tunnel's opening. Think of a train backing in and out of a railroad tunnel with one car that is about an inch taller than the tunnel—grinding, screeching, lurching.

The mechanical mismatch in trigger finger is greatest in the morning after the thickened area has had all night to swell up. Patients usually notice that the locking loosens up as they begin to use their hands. Warm water helps.

What else can be done? Several treatment efforts may be required to obtain relief. First, a long-acting cortisone preparation is injected into the tunnel to reduce the tendon's swelling. About half of trigger fingers respond completely and permanently to this injection. If relief is incomplete, a second injection one month later is advisable.

For the small percentage of trigger fingers not responsive to two injections, a short outpatient surgical procedure under local anesthesia works well. The roof of the tunnel is opened slightly to give the thickened tendon ample gliding room. Sometimes over a number of years, individuals may need treatment for nearly all their fingers. The good news is that nobody gets trigger toes.

OH, MY ACHING THUMB

With several garden projects in mind, I collected a huge stack of used brick after the 1994 Northridge earthquake. Neighbors dumped debris from their damaged chimneys at curbside pending removal. I spent many 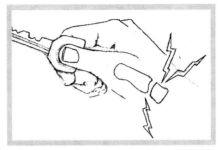 evenings retrieving whole bricks, holding them in one hand while hammering the mortar off, then stacking them in the station wagon and stacking them again at home. After a while, the base of my brick-holding thumb began hurting. It has never completely recovered.

I thereby joined the ranks of people over 45 who have an ache at the base of their thumbs with forceful pinching and gripping activities— such as opening jars, lifting heavy books, shaking hands, turning keys, pulling on tight clothes. What is going on?

The joint where the thumb connects to the wrist is quite 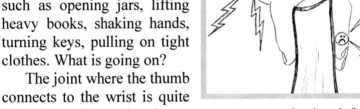 flexible. It allows thumb movement across the hand for fixing buttons, away from the palm for grasping milk cartons, and lying flat next to the index finger for crawling or clapping. The joint is also strong. When we pinch with 15 pounds of force to turn a tight key, about 125 pounds of force is generated at the thumb's base. After 40-50 years of vigorous use, this joint begins to slip slightly out of place and ache from wear and tear—osteoarthritis. The good news is that the thumb's versatility and its connections to a big brain have allowed for eons of extensive tool use and civilization building. The bad news is that our remarkable thumbs can wear out long before the rest of us does. For uncertain reasons, pain usually starts earlier in the non-dominant thumb and may never affect the dominant thumb.

Several other reassurances are in order. First, getting osteoarthritis in the thumb is by no means a prelude to having generalized gnarling of fingers, hips, and knees. Second, treatment is helpful.

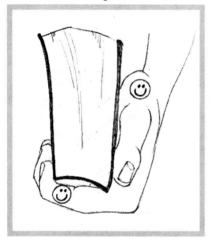

Of foremost importance is to stop abusing the aching joint. This means stop using it for forceful pinch where possible. This is hard, because these use patterns are deeply ingrained after 40-50 years of pain-free use, and it is hard to get through the day without using our thumbs. Learn to grasp books and heavy files from below, lubricate locks to make keys easier to turn, and use a dandelion digger to loosen weeds before pulling them. Use a gadget for tight bottle caps and jar lids. A hand therapist can make a custom-molded plastic brace that supports and protects the ailing joint while allowing for nearly full hand function. It also reminds the user to find alternate, pain-free ways of doing things. After wearing the brace for six to eight weeks, the pain generally subsides and may stay away for months. Then an episode of kneading bread or moving books may stir it up again, in which case the brace goes back on for a while. The brace is the only treatment many people ever need.

If the arthritis progresses to the point that tearing open envelopes or brushing teeth becomes a daily ordeal, then surgery can help. Several surgical procedures are available. The best seems to be removal of the sugar cube-sized arthritic wrist bone at the thumb's base, then restoring the thumb to its original position and holding it there for the first five weeks with a steel pin and cast. During that time, the space vacated by the small bone fills with scar tissue, which has three beneficial features. The scar becomes strong enough to withstand fully forceful pinch. The scar can become sufficiently flexible to restore full thumb motion. The scar does not have any nerve fibers, so the pain goes away. By four months after surgery, nearly all patients are gleefully back to full activity.

I have a brace. I need it and wear it less than a week a year now. The ache is mild and intermittent, does not limit my activities, and allows me to relate to patients who have the same problem. Should I eventually require surgery, those bricks may turn out to be expensive.

GLUCOSAMINE AND CHONDROITIN FOR ARTHRITIS

Is there a scientific basis for oral glucosamine and chondroitin sulfate rebuilding cartilage in arthritic joints? Are these expensive pills the miracle cure we have been waiting for? The answer to both questions, sadly, is no.

The cartilage surfacing our joints is a huge, complex molecular mesh that has chondroitin sulfate and glucosamine as two of its building blocks. Since they are broken down into small, basic molecules in the digestive system after being swallowed, these pills are no more beneficial to the joints than eating a balanced diet.

As you might suspect, eating brain does not make one smarter, nor does swallowing bones make one's fracture heal faster. The same is true for cartilage. Hype, fad, and placebo effect account for any benefits reported. No scientifically valid study supports their use. Furthermore, the government considers glucosamine and chondroitin sulfate to be dietary supplements rather than drugs, and neither the U.S. Food and Drug Administration nor any other watchdog regulates their purity. The fact that the bottle label says "Glucosamine" or "Chondroitin Sulfate" means little. Yes, some people swear by these supplements, and they probably won't hurt you other than in your pocketbook. Just ask yourself, though: Does eating hair cure baldness?

Now that we have looked at some of the common disorders that affect our hands through life, we will turn to an issue that affects our hands on a daily basis—work.

3

HANDS
At Work

A BOUT 2500 YEARS AGO, THE ETRUSCANS, UNDER THE leadership of King Porsenna, besieged Rome. In an effort to end the siege and save his city, a Roman youth, Caius Mucius, sought and received permission to sneak into the enemy camp and kill Porsenna. Once in the Etruscan court he could not clearly identify the king and was smart not to ask. Instead he killed the best-dressed man there, who unfortunately turned out to be the king's secretary.

Captured and brought before Porsenna, Mucius remained undaunted. He calmly told the king that he was just an ordinary Roman citizen and that any Roman would duplicate his act to protect their beloved city. Then Mucius demonstrated his sincerity and indifference to suffering by placing his right hand in an altar fire and letting it burn without flinching.

Dazzled by this show of bravery, Porsenna released Mucius. In return for the king's mercy, Mucius revealed that he was merely the first of 300 Romans sworn to kill Porsenna and that all were equally committed. The king, intimidated by this (false) information, decided to negotiate a peace with the Romans rather than risk his life to enemies as loyal and determined as Mucius. On his return to Rome, Mucius became known as Scaevola ("left-handed") and was rewarded a tract of land near his beloved city.

Maybe we would not voluntarily destroy our hands for society the way Scaevola did, but hands have been integral workplace tools throughout history. When ancestral man first stood up, hands were used to hunt and gather, later to plant seeds, and then to make and use tools. When language came about, our ancient ancestors probably called hunting, gathering, farming, and tool fabrication *survival*. Today we call them occupations and our hands are indispensable for nearly all means of employment. Here is a spectrum of ways hands do work (beyond intimidating kings), how they can get injured in the process, some ways to protect them, and two extraordinary ways hands work to combat deafness and blindness.

OF MICE AND GLADIATORS

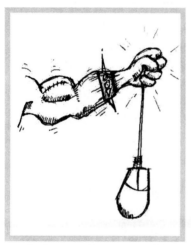

In an old gladiator movie, the imprisoned hero is commanded to hold a fist-sized rock out at arm's length. "No problem," the handsome brute smirks. But after a while, this simple task turns into an impossible feat as the warrior's muscles melt into quivering jelly.

The modern day equivalent of this tortuous lesson in humility is, believe it or not, the computer mouse. Especially when used intensely and for prolonged periods—such as scrolling through data or drawing intricate diagrams—the mouse can affect every living cell from fingertip to neck. If you don't believe that contracting a muscle and then not moving it much can make you hurt, forcefully hold your fingers as if they were grasping a grapefruit while you read this section.

Too much time with a mouse is one way to get overuse syndrome. Tendons, muscles, nerves, and joint capsules become achy and sore when touched, first just while mousing, then for progressively longer periods after the offending mouse has been fingered and caged. If not attended to, the ache can last for months. The debility can extend to basic activities such as fastening buttons and brushing teeth.

Why do certain computer gladiators get overuse syndrome while their coworkers and neighbors may not? It is probably related to subtle physiological and anatomical differences, the same type of differences that allow some lucky individuals to sing beautifully and others to high jump seven feet. Some people can mouse with impunity, but the rest of us, including anybody whose hand is now aching from holding the imaginary grapefruit, have limitations. If you are a workaholic, have a type A personality, are stressed from an impending deadline, and play video games for "relaxation" when you finally drag yourself home at 10 pm, you are more likely to develop overuse syndrome. As the flight commander tells Maverick in *Top Gun*, "Your ego is writing checks that your body can't cash."

Overuse syndrome is best avoided. If you mouse a lot and have ever noted your hand aching, pay close attention. First, get an alternate control device—a trackball or touch pad for instance. Then alternate your mouse *and* the new control between both hands. (For the severely impaired, foot-controlled mice are also available.) The various controllers require use of different muscles, and the goal is to rotate the workload on an hourly basis among many muscles in both hands. Think of it this way. Which is better, hopping all the way to the store on one leg or walking uphill and cycling down?

As for the computer keyboard, it should be directly in front of you and at a height where your forearms are parallel to the floor with your hands projecting straight ahead on your forearms. For people of average height this means lowering their keyboard below standard desk height or raising their chair. To do otherwise unnecessarily stresses and fatigues the finger-controlling tendons as they cross the wrist. The fatigued tendons in turn can press on adjacent nerves and joint capsules. All sorts of information-age agonies can ensue, but the history of overuse goes back to the industrial age.

A hundred years ago, overuse syndrome was epidemic among telegraphers. Then their problem (and their job) suddenly disappeared with the development of the telephone and radio. Typewriters came along and people learned to put them on deskside typing tables, which lowered the typewriter's keyboard so that the operators' wrists were appropriately positioned. Slapping the carriage return, inserting new sheets of paper, and manually correcting errors gave the fingers time to rest as well as providing the shoulder and elbow muscles a little exercise. All was well.

Then computers arrived. We plopped the keyboard on top of the desk, placed our wrists in awkward positions, and started pounding relentlessly. Ache, ache, ache. A hundred years from now, we will control our computers by voice or telepathy, and "mouse-itis" will be as rare as gladiator shoulder. In the meantime, respect those electronic pain makers on your desk. Helpful information about computer positioning and use is available at healthycomputing.com.

STOCKBROKER'S ELBOW

Sitting at a desk can be perilous even if there are no mice in sight. Nearly everyone has heard of carpal tunnel syndrome—pressure on a major nerve at the wrist that causes tingling and numbness in the thumb, index, and middle fingers, especially at night. A slightly less common but equally irksome problem is cubital tunnel syndrome. *Cubitus* is Latin for elbow, and through this enclosed channel on the inside of your elbow runs the ulnar nerve. It is your funny bone.

When the ulnar nerve is squeezed at the elbow, its blood supply is cut off and it responds by causing numbness and tingling in

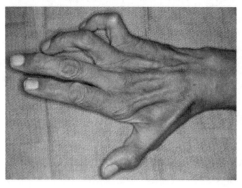

the ring and small fingers. This happens occasionally, especially at night, to most of us, and usually we change position and it goes away. If the pressure remains constant or occurs repeatedly over weeks, the numbness becomes constant and the small muscles in the hand that contribute greatly to digital strength and dexterity become weak. The hand in the figure demonstrates advanced cubital tunnel syndrome where the small muscles have wasted away and the individual is no longer able to extend his ring and small fingers fully.

Cubital tunnel syndrome usually develops for no explainable reason, but it certainly can be made worse by leaving the elbow completely bent—especially if the elbow and the ulnar nerve rest on a hard surface, such as on a desktop while using a telephone. Therefore stockbrokers, telephone solicitors, and receptionists are particularly at risk.

Everybody has a hand or foot go to sleep occasionally, and that is not a problem; but if your ring and little finger tingle every day, then treatment is in order. Treatment reduces pressure on the nerve, by nonoperative means if possible.

People who live on the phone should use a headset for hands-free yakking. During the day, everyone should avoid prolonged elbow pressure against the armrests on their desk chair and in their car. At work, change chairs or take the armrests off and in your car flip the armrest up so you won't be tempted to compress the nerve. If that brute next to you on the airplane is hogging the armrest, comfort yourself with the awareness that he will get cubital tunnel syndrome and you won't!

At night, position yourself in bed with your elbows straight or nearly straight. This minimizes pressure on the nerve and helps it recover from the day's insults. If you actually want to get some sleep and not worry all night about your elbow position, make a soft splint with a bath towel and safety pins. Start by folding the sides of the towel over so that it is as wide as your arm is long from armpit to wrist, then roll the towel around your arm to make a tube and safety pin this tube together. At bedtime slip this thick sleeve onto your arm. It is bulky enough to prevent your elbow from closing much even after you fall asleep and blissfully return to the curled up fetal position.

If symptoms persist despite avoiding direct pressure and keeping your elbow straight day and night, early surgery generally yields good recovery. Operations take the pressure off the nerve either by making the tunnel larger or by moving the nerve out of the tunnel. Any of these surgical treatments can usually be performed on an outpatient basis with some sedation while numbing just the arm. Within a day or two, self-care and desk-type activities are possible, and strenuous elbow activities such as tennis, yoga, or push-ups can follow in about six weeks.

Delayed treatment risks permanent weakness for pinch and grip activities such as turning keys and holding steering wheels, which leads us to another peril of the machine age, the car itself.

HAND SAFETY IN THE CAR

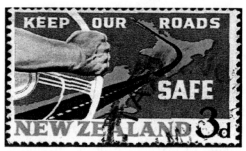

Carl Benz may have sustained the first automobile accident ever. During an 1885 public display of his invention, he forgot to steer and crashed into a wall. In the intervening years, deaths and injuries from automobile accidents have been, unfortunately, too common. Each decade, however, has seen refinements for improved safety to life and limb, including hands.

For instance, a common injury, known as the chauffeur's fracture, resulted from the starting crank kicking back and breaking the operator's wrist. Electric starters eliminated that risk. More recently, headrests have minimized whiplash injuries to the neck and the associated pinched nerves.

Air conditioning is at least partially responsible for eliminating the particularly gruesome sideswipe injury. In this situation a driver's left elbow and forearm, resting on the open window ledge, would be struck by a closely passing vehicle. Wider roads also get some credit for reducing this characteristic left-sided injury.

Unfortunately, doctors still see hand injuries resulting when people travel in cars with open windows. In roll-over accidents, an occupant may reflexively put his hand outside the window and on the car's roof in an effort to support himself. The hand then gets trapped between the car's roof and the ground. To avoid such out-of-car risks, leave the window next to you completely or at least nearly closed.

Other serious dangers lurk *inside* the car. Here lap-shoulder belts and air bags help protect occupants from life-threatening contact with the steering wheel, dashboard, and windshield. Used in combination, these restraint systems reduce the risk of fatality by half during head-on accidents. Their lifesaving effectiveness is proven, and driver and front passenger air bags became standard equipment on all new cars in 1998.

Air bags, however, pose a risk to hands and forearms. Air bag inflation is by necessity a very rapid and forceful event, occurring in one-tenth of a second at a velocity estimated between 150 and 200 miles per hour. When the driver's hands are inside the steering wheel, the inflating bag can force the hands against the wheel with sufficient force to break bones. For an extra bit of air bag safety, hold the wheel on the outside, and never reach through the steering wheel to adjust the car's controls or to rest your hands.

Despite many remarkable refinements since Carl Benz's time, no innovation is even on the horizon to protect us from the most common automotive risk to hands. Only awareness of and respect for car doors, hoods, and trunk lids can keep fingertips safe. The good news about car doors is that they are engineered to have enough give that they rarely do serious damage to trapped fingertips. One unfortunate patient of mine, however, dropped her keys as she locked her fingertip in the door. She had an agonizing wait until somebody came by, retrieved her keys, and freed her insulted finger.

So if you think that the tools in the office and the cars that get us there are hard on hands, read on. Sharpened steel has no conscience whatsoever.

TOOL SAFETY

I recall deeply gouging my palm with a chisel when I was a teenager. It was dull and so I was pushing hard, and my other hand was in the chisel's trajectory. I still look at the scar and think how that needless injury could have been career defining for me. Fortunately the chisel missed my tendons and nerves, so limitations of motion and sensation were not restraints when I decided on hand surgery.

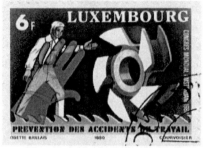

Unfortunately, not all my patients have been as lucky. Even use of the simplest tools such as kitchen knives (more on them in Chapter 6), craft knives, and screwdrivers can result in permanent stiffness and numbness. It is truly a small expense to have a range of sharp, good-quality tools compared with the cost of emergency care and the risk of permanent damage to your hand. Avoid those six-in-one and fifty-in-one all-purpose gadgets. A tool designed to perform multiple tasks is unlikely to do any of them well. Treat every tool in your utility drawer, toolbox, or workshop with the respect divers give sharks--all are effective, some are harmless, and a few are potentially lethal.

Many accidents happen when the user is mentally or physically off balance. Fatigue, anger, and haste—as well as standing precariously, not securing the work, and using tools for unintended purposes—are formulas for disaster.

You have to push harder to power a dull craft knife or an old, rounded screwdriver, so when you lose control the steel edge is going to go farther, faster. Even when the tool is sharp, imagine where it might go should it slip, and then keep your hand out of that zone. And, think where your hand might go if it slips off the tool or the work. For instance, experienced mechanics will use a wrench by pulling it toward them rather than pushing on it. If the wrench slips off the nut, the pusher's fist strikes the first available solid object, while the puller's fist comes back safely toward the body.

If you have ever had a hammer glance off a nail and mar your work or your thumb, try sharpening it. Rubbing the face of the hammer with sandpaper produces a nonskid surface. It does not last long but is easy to renew. For you power nailers, remember that a nail gun may remain pressurized and dangerous even after the pneumatic hose has been disconnected. Every hand surgeon has taken a few power-driven nails out of carpenters' hands.

Power saws are the "great whites" of the workshop. Much of the blade is concealed, but the uncaring teeth are coming toward you at roughly 100 miles per hour. Anger and haste are shark bait, so take a break until you can focus on the dangers. All adjustments and blade replace-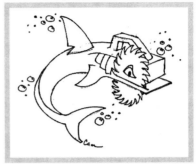
ments are wisely done with the motor unplugged. It's an awkward nuisance to use the blade guard and a push stick, but before bypassing them, imagine being gnawed by a shark. Also, adjust the blade exposure so that the blade just barely clears the work, then at least any injury will be from a small shark.

Electric handsaws are the ultimate danger. Should the blade bind for any reason, the entire whirling machine kicks out of the work and viciously lunges toward the operator. The hand holding the work is at extreme risk. When I talk to people who have sustained injuries with an electric handsaw, they commonly describe one of three scenarios: knots, nails, and knees. The first two can obviously stop the blade moving forward and send the whole saw flying backward. In the third instance, the operator is holding the work over his knee, and as the cut is nearing completion, the board bends and binds the blade. Calamity ensues.

I hope I have persuaded you to visit the hardware store soon. If you don't know a feather board from a miter box, at least pick up a new screwdriver and a pack of replacement blades for your craft knife. If you are into *This Old House*, get all your blades sharpened and invest in some sawhorses. Either way, when you get down to work, respect the sharks.

A SAW WITH A CONSCIENCE

Since their invention, power saws have had a taste for fingers. That is now changing. A physicist/woodworker has invented a device that is now available on new table saws, adding perhaps $50-100 to the cost of the saw but vastly improving its safety.

Circuitry in the new saw senses the blade's electrical environment. Wood, even wet wood, has little capacity to store electricity. The saw runs. The human body is 90% water and has a large capacity to store electricity. When a saw tooth touches skin, the blade senses an electrical change and stops dead within 5/1000th of a second. That is before it can make a third of a revolution.

Check out the website, SawStop.com. It includes a video clip of a sacrificial hotdog being pushed into a table saw. The hotdog barely gets nicked before the saw stops. Craftsmen's fingers will be spared, as will hotdogs.

MOWERS AND BLOWERS

Lawnmowers and snowblowers quite efficiently remove and eject anything in their paths. Unfortunately, this includes fingertips. We are probably smarter than the man who tried trimming his hedge by holding his lawnmower over it, but every year tens of thousands of injuries occur from less obvious misuse of these laborsaving machines.

Water is the principal factor that causes both snowblowers and lawnmowers to clog and then to beckon for a helping hand. Wet, heavy snow on a warm day easily blocks the exit chute. This snowball conceals the proximity and awesome power of the spinning blades. Wet grass clippings do the same. The obvious advice is to shut the machine down before removing the obstruction. Haste makes waste.

Snowblowers offer a special surprise because the impeller blades continue to spin, unseen and barely heard, for several seconds after the motor stops completely. Shut it down, then take five seconds to admire the beauty of the day and your intact gloves before relieving the blockage. Even then, use a stick or rolled-up newspaper to explore the unknown. The only good news about snowblower injuries is that they rarely get infected. Snow is clean.

By contrast, grass is filthy and the myriad microorganisms contaminating a fingertip injury greatly enhance the risk of infection and amputation. Lawnmowers confer some other risks. Resist the temptation to give a child a ride. Wear closed-toed shoes. Follow the manufacturer's advice precisely when mowing slopes because slipping under a push mower or having a riding mower roll over on top of you is not a pretty thought.

I could go on about the catalysts of alcohol, foiled safety shields and dead-man switches, and use of the mower to trim hedges or the blower to clean your child's room, but these warnings are in the owner's manual. I will, however, give you permission to go inside and just wait for the snow to melt and the grass to dry.

The battlefield is an even more dangerous environment for hands than driveways and lawns are. It was from an awareness of such injuries during World War II that hand surgery developed as a distinct specialty.

EXACTLY WHAT IS HAND SURGERY?

Compared to cardiac surgery or neurology, which are medical specialties focused on a particular organ (the heart) or a particular tissue (nerves), hand surgery is a regional specialty. During World War II, for the first time, many soldiers with major injuries survived but then required complex limb reconstruction for burns, shrapnel injuries, and amputations.

The U.S. Surgeon General recognized that having a series of tissue specialists line up first to fix the hand's skeleton (orthopedist), then the nerves (neurosurgeon), then the arteries (vascular surgeon), then tendons and then skin (plastic surgeon) was obviously impractical. He appointed a general surgeon friend of his from San Francisco, one of perhaps five doctors in the country at that time who specialized in surgery of the hand, to train a cadre of military surgeons and to develop hand surgery as a specialty.

From that beginning, hand surgeons learned to manage all of the hand's unique tissues in concert. This regional approach clearly offers the best opportunity to restore the hand to its maximal function and appearance. Just at the end of World War II, this small group organized the American Society for Surgery of the Hand, which has grown to over 2000 hand surgery specialists in the ensuing decades.

What is a hand surgeon's territory? The hand, wrist, and forearm are always included; and depending on the doctor's background and interest, he or she may possibly treat elbow and shoulder problems as well as the nerves passing from the neck into the arm.

To train in hand surgery, a medical school graduate (four years after college) first completes residency training in orthopedic, plastic, or general surgery (five to seven years) and then takes an additional year of fellowship training to learn the nuances of treating all the tissues affecting the hand. Several years after becoming board certified in orthopedic, plastic, or general surgery, the aspiring hand surgeon can then sit for another rigorous examination to obtain the Certificate of Added Qualifications in Surgery of the Hand. This certificate, which requires renewal by examination every 10 years, recognizes true specialists in treating this functionally and aesthetically important body region.

Even so, when I tell new acquaintances that I am a hand surgeon they frequently respond with a quizzical look, pause, and ask, "Is that all you do?" They have difficulty imagining how I could possibly stay busy restricting my practice to such a limited anatomical area, especially if they have never encountered a hand problem themselves. Here is a brief breakdown of what I do at work all day. I treat three fourths of the patients I see with some combination of rest, reassurance, medications, splints/casts, and activity modification. Year in and year out, I average more than one operation a day—one of roughly 300 different procedures. Three fourths of the operations are for "acquired" conditions. These include nerve compressions such as carpal tunnel syndrome, tendonitis, and tumors. The other fourth are mostly for injuries, both recent and old, with a small remainder of operations for treatment of infections or congenital abnormalities. Of the roughly 2000 American hand surgeons, some are busier treating patients than I am, others are less busy treating patients but spend more time evaluating them for workers' compensation.

I think hand surgery may be more challenging than most other surgical specialties. I say this not from a technical point of view, because surgeons, some of them with sizeable egos, could argue themselves blue about whether it is more difficult to remove a brain tumor, replant a finger, or revascularize a heart. Rather I say hand surgery is more challenging because most of us have two hands and ten fingers in plain sight. Naturally curious, we compare them. Then if one is bandaged, it readily attracts comment from other people, who recount their own experiences. So perhaps more challenging, yes; but perhaps more rewarding as well? Also yes, and for the same reason. The hand surgeon's work is exposed for all to see, and many times the resultant deviations from normal are sufficiently subtle that nobody notices. Most satisfying.

PICKING POCKETS

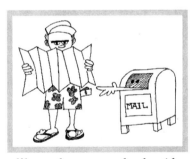

Pockets are wonderful creations, made by hands and useful for hands, yet we give them little thought until somebody else's hand has been inside to swipe our wallet. So in order to pay respect to the oft ignored pocket, here's how picking pockets works.

Distractions are a good tactic—like when somebody (the stall) stops abruptly in front of you (the mark) on the sidewalk and then somebody else (the pick) bumps forcefully into you from behind because of your (you presume) unpredictable stop. You apologize, brush yourself off and only later realize that your billfold is missing. You made it easy by having it in your hip pocket (the sucker's pocket), especially if the pants are loose. Even an amateur can do it when the pocket is left unbuttoned. Somebody can think about only so much at once, and the bump distracts you from everything else. A more elaborate distraction, which may even allow picking a jacket pocket, is when somebody "accidentally" spills ice cream on you and then graciously(!) and vigorously helps you clean it off.

Crowds are also good. The dip and accomplice(s) can quickly find easy marks, they can quickly fade away if detected, and jostling is the norm. Big crowds are even better--bodies pressed together at turnstiles or on subways for instance. Zippers on fanny packs and backpacks are child's play when the dip is behind you. The preferred technique is to reach across with his or her far hand when standing beside you while that forearm is innocently covered with a newspaper or jacket. Rather than reaching deep into your pocket, the expert deftly brings folds of the pocket into his fingers to raise the prize to the surface. Once lifted, he immediately passes your goods to an accomplice, so if you should finger the dip, he is clean.

Pickpockets hate people who distribute their valuables among various pockets or wear money belts. Other dislikes include tight pants, front pockets, wallets with rubber bands around them or with combs wedged inside, and purses with zipped zippers and snapped snaps. Should you be robbed, don't oblige the dip by shouting, "Pickpocket!" If you do, everybody nearby will instinctively pat his wallet, tipping the dip to its location. Even when pickpockets have successfully extracted your wallet, they get upset if you left your credit cards and big bills at home.

Here is one last thought about ice cream. One night the ticket taker at a movie would not allow me to enter until I had finished my cone of nut fudge ripple. Rather than miss the opening scene, I went around the corner, wrapped my unfinished dessert in a couple of paper napkins, slipped it into the front pocket of my relaxed-fit khakis and walked in. I was kind of hoping that the person in front of me would suddenly stop and that I would get bumped from behind. The dip would not find cold cash but cold cashew fudge ripple.

TIPS FOR THE BOSS

Imagine workplace loyalty so fierce that when you err you seek forgiveness by cutting off the last segment of your little finger. Then you wrap the part in fine cloth and solemnly offer it to your boss. This age-old ritual amputation, *yubitsume*, is practiced by the yakuza, Japan's equivalent of the Mafia.

In addition to organizing crime units in families, the Japanese yakuza have a unique arrangement known as *oyabun/kobun*— father role/child role. The oyabun advises and nurtures, and in return the kobun provides unwavering loyalty and service whenever needed. The loyalty, trust, and obedience so engendered can lead to a fanatic devotion to the boss. The kobun takes the bullet or the rap as necessary to protect his mentor.

Yubitsume began hundreds of years ago as a means of dealing with serious infractions that did not quite warrant death or expulsion. With a weakened hand, the kobun could not grip his all-important sword as firmly as before. Thus, a warrior so disciplined became more dependent on the protection of his boss. Subsequent infractions could result in amputation at the second joint of the same finger or at the last joint of another finger. As a reminder that the gang's policies were not to be ignored, the severed fingers, preserved in alcohol, were prominently displayed at headquarters.

Traditionally, the yakuza has operated much more openly than the organized underworld in America. A Japanese government-sponsored survey in the 1970s found that 42% of yakuza members sported short pinkie fingers. Together with full-body tattoos, these amputations have symbolized machismo and willingness to endure pain for the benefit of the organization. This seems to be changing, however, as the Japanese public grows less tolerant of and less intimidated by the yakuza. An anti-gangster law passed in 1992 has also helped. Many yakuza have had to go straight to make a living, and any external sign of their former criminal life is a detriment.

Some former members have had slip-on silicone rubber pinkies made. The naturally appearing prosthesis costs a minimum of $3000 yet provides no movement or sensation. A ring, though, can completely hide the junction where the realistic-appearing substitute fits over the finger stump. A little dirt under the nail heightens the deception. It is too soon to tell what the availability of lifelike finger substitutes will have on yubitsume.

Maybe a repeat offender can just offer the boss his prosthesis rather than the real thing.

HANDS THAT TALK, HANDS THAT HEAR

Adorning conversation with hand gestures is common in various cultures around the world and virtually obligatory in some, but communicating with hand gestures alone occurs more often than you may think. Various forms of manual communication are used not only by deaf individuals and their acquaintances, but also by divers, crane operators, flight line personnel, and factory workers when communication by sound presents problems.

Manual communication comes in several forms. Finger spelling uses a distinct finger position to represent each letter and number. It is easy to learn, slow to use, but valuable for introduction of new names or difficult concepts into a conversation.

Signed English is faster and is a direct translation of spoken English into signs. Here the signer presents each word visually and in the same sequence as speech. People who become deaf later in life often use Signed English.

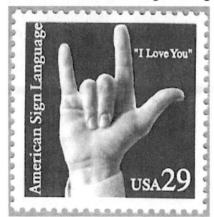

American Sign Language (ASL) is a distinct language with its own grammar, subtleties, and richness especially suited to the capabilities of the hands and eyes. Manual puns come easily, and some say that ASL is even more expressive than English. Not only does the shape of the hands impart meaning, but so does their beginning and ending locations in front of the face or chest. Signers shout by making large, brisk signs, or they can make small, partially concealed signs if they do not want their conversation to be 'overseen.'

Individuals who are deaf from birth or from an early age often prefer ASL. Hearing infants who are signed to from birth will often use signs themselves long before they develop intelligible speech. After English and Spanish, ASL and Italian vie for the third most commonly used language in the United States.

How do deaf individuals with injured or deformed hands talk? I asked myself that question, queried my deaf patients, did a survey, and learned some interesting things. Absent digits, stiff joints, or weak muscles may result in looser signing patterns but do not cause much loss of meaning—similar to the difficulties caused in written communication by poor penmanship or in conversation by hoarseness or a heavy accent.

Sign language interpreters are hearing individuals who translate when deaf persons and hearing nonsigners need to communicate in a classroom, courtroom, or doctor's office, for instance. Like vocal cords, which tire after prolonged speech, limb muscles in signers deserve protection from overuse. Warm-up exercises and frequent breaks with stretching exercises are helpful. Interpreters can also diminish their need for tiresome finger spelling by increasing their signing vocabulary. Particularly taxing for interpreters is signing for an individual who is both deaf and blind and who feels the signs rather than sees them. This is truly hand-to-hand communication.

HANDS THAT READ

Louis Braille, blind from age 3, devised a system of raised dots in groups of six to represent letters and numbers. By the time he was 20, he had perfected this system for tactile reading. For the ensuing 180 years, blind and severely visually impaired people have read this way. Later embellishments in notation allowed braille users to read music and mathematical formulas. Now, iPods, audio books, talking computers, and other high-tech innovations have replaced braille for some purposes, but similar electronic technologies have also made braille more useful in other settings, meaning that braille is not going away. It will be worthwhile learning a little about how people read with their hands.

Each braille cell, almost an eighth of an inch wide and less than a fourth of an inch high, has six dots. Braille letters are made by raising one or more dots in the cell so that an experienced fingertip passing over them can detect meaning. For instance, one dot in the upper left corner of the cell represents *a* and three vertical dots in a row represents *l*. Sixty-three dot combinations are possible, so all letters are represented along with punctuation marks and certain common words, such as *and, for,* and *the,* and certain commonly occurring letter combinations, such as *ch, th,* and *er.* Numerals 0-9 are represented by the same dot patterns that represent letters a through j; but when a number is meant, it is preceded by a special dot pattern that says what follows is a number rather than a letter. Another dot combination alerts the reader that the next letter is capitalized. Dot combinations also identify each musical note on the scale along with its timing -- an eighth note or a quarter note for instance. Braille can also clearly represent rests, accidentals, and every other notation in music. The same goes for mathematical formulas and bookkeeping accounts.

Braille users have their own personal styles for passing their fingers over the rows of cells. Many use their right index finger to actually do the reading while their right small finger scouts ahead and their left index finger identifies the next line. Speed greatly increases when a reader advances from uncontracted to contracted braille. Here 189 contractions and abbreviations reduce the number of cells needed to express a word. For instance in contracted braille, *brl* means braille and *k* means knowledge. Thus, the same symbol can mean several different things depending on its position in a word and sentence, so the context is important.

Of course, braille can be written as well as read. The writer places a heavy sheet of paper between a hinged plastic or metal "slate" that has the cells punched out. A pointed stylus can then be used to raise dots on the opposite side of the paper. A braille eraser has a blunt tip to flatten a raised dot.

Commercially, braille can be printed on both sides of a sheet of paper by aligning (interpointing) the cells and rows such that the raised dots on one side fall between the raised dots on the other side. Standard-sized braille paper is 11 inches square, and three braille pages approximate one conventionally printed page. Thus, braille books are bulky. Tolkien's *The Fellowship of the Ring* is seven volumes of interpoint braille. Alternatively, now people can carry all of Tolkien's work plus hundreds of songs and today's newspaper around in an iPod and listen to any of it without spreading out a big braille book on their lap. So why is braille still important?

For one thing, scanning text in electronic media is awkward and comprehending spatially arranged information such as music and data spreadsheets is nearly impossible. Second, modern technology has made braille more versatile. Electronic braille writers have streamlined writing over what is possible with a slate and stylus. A braillewriter is somewhat like a typewriter, but essentially with six keys (one for each dot position in a cell) and a space bar. Then for reading, a braille terminal is a device that has several rows of cells with six pins in each cell that form dots when raised. Therefore, a book can be downloaded electronically, stored, and presented two lines at a time.

Similarly, a device known as a screen reader can pass words on a computer screen through a speaker to create audible speech or through the braille terminal to provide tactile appreciation of the message. Smaller, portable versions of braille terminals, called note takers, have 18-40 cells and are useful for quickly jotting reminders and reviewing them later. Braille terminals and note takers are expensive because each tiny pin in each cell has to function perfectly. For example, if the pin in the upper left corner of a cell malfunctioned, an *a* would be turned into a space.

Isn't braille fascinating? When I see those combinations of dots in elevators and taxicabs, I run my finger over them. I am lucky if I can tell where one cell stops and the next one starts. With practice, I am told, the meaning comes clear. Way to go, fingertips.

HANDS THAT WORK NOT QUITE RIGHT

Its medical name is focal dystonia. Tailors can get it. Writers and artists call it writer's cramps. Golfers call it the yips.

Musicians at times have to call it quits when they get a focal dystonia, which is an incompletely understood movement disorder where the brain gives a particular muscle or muscle group a slightly altered message about the timing and power of contraction.

On a musical instrument, a finger may curl under when the musician wants it straight, or it may mysteriously straighten out when the musician tries to curl it. Putters, pens, and brushes seem to have minds of their own. Scott Adams, after successfully drawing Dilbert cartoons for over 15 years, discovered that he could no longer draw a straight line. Every time he tried, his little finger would go rigidly straight when he wanted it bent. He tried various medical treatments and even tried drawing left-handed before getting around the problem by cartooning on a large computer tablet where unaffected shoulder muscles could adequately control the stylus. Such a change of technique is often the only answer, but this is difficult or impossible in some situations.

The renowned pianist Leon Fleisher had his career side-tracked by a focal dystonia in his right ring and small fingers. After multiple failed treatments, he resorted to playing music written solely for the left hand, and in recent years he has noted some improvement in his right hand following Botox injections. This naturally occurring toxin paralyzes nearby muscles for a matter of months, but the balance between too little and too much is extremely narrow, especially for those people who rely on the finest motor movements to perfect their work.

Focal dystonia is usually task-specific, meaning that dexterity is normal for all other activities. Let's look next at hands that have more obvious departures from normal and affect every aspect of their owners' lives.

CHAPTER

4

HANDS

With Differences

A SEVEN-YEAR OLD GIRL—LET'S CALL HER JULIE—AND her mom and grandmother came to see me in the office one day. The exam room was quiet when I walked in, but they were having an animated conversation—in sign language. When she was listening and wasn't signing, I could count Julie's fingers, six fingers on one hand and seven on the other, but no thumbs. Through the sign language interpreter, I learned that the family was there to have this rare congenital difference addressed so that Julie could more easily hold a pen, tie her shoes, and do the other things thumbs are good for. I explained that I could remove the extra digits, which would leave normal small, ring, middle, and two index fingers on both hands. I recommended then shortening and rotating the outside index fingers to make thumbs. The interpreter commented that these corrections would also likely make Julie's signing easier to understand.

The operations were successful. Not only was Julie's ability to use her hands for everyday tasks markedly better, she could now sign clearly even to strangers and casual acquaintances. I realized that this was my one chance as a hand surgeon to correct a speech impediment. More broadly, it reminds me of the ways people can find their way in life by extraordinary use of their hands, even though they may be different from yours and mine.

INDIVIDUAL VARIATION

Pale. Slender. Stocky. Grizzled. Pudgy. Robust. These words can describe people's appearances, and such variations allow us to recognize each other. Without these differences we would have to ask, "Are you Joe or Bill?" How dull and confusing it would be if everyone looked alike.

The words listed above also describe peoples' hands, and in fact, we could probably recognize many of our friends and family by seeing just their hands. What is unknown to most people, however, is that the differences in hands do not stop at the skin. Hand surgeons expect and savor internal variation. It makes each hand special. Let's peek inside.

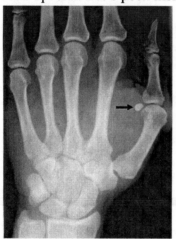

When somebody asks me how many bones there are in the hand, I respond honestly, "I don't know." The textbook answer is 27, but nearly everybody has a few extra little bones, and occasionally the wrist will have seven bones rather than eight. So without looking at an individual's x-rays, I really can't say for sure.

Here is an example that you can see from the surface. Bend your thumb across your palm as far as it will go. Look at the second joint back from the tip. From person to person there is more variability in this joint than anyplace else in the body. Some people can bend it 90 degrees, others can barely bend it at all. When examining an injury to the area, a

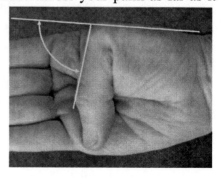

hand surgeon has to decide if the observed stiffness is related to the injury or if it is just the way that individual was assembled. A check of the opposite thumb is helpful, since these joints are usually the same in both hands.

The same holds true for the alignment of our fingers, which are usually a little crooked, even in the absence of injury or arthritis. If your left little finger has a bow in it, your right little finger is probably a mirror image. In other instances, left to right differences are possible.

Take for example a specific tendon at your wrist. Look for it

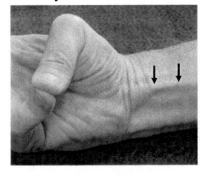

by firmly pushing the tips of your thumb and your small finger together and bending your palm toward your forearm. Usually a tendon right in the middle jumps up and tents the skin, but it is absent in roughly one out of seven hands. It may be present on one side and missing on the other.

How about nerves? Sensation to each finger comes from one of two major nerves, except for the ring finger, which usually gets its sensation from both, but not always. The same is true for those fleshy muscles at the base of your thumb. One nerve supplies most of them, but crossovers from another nerve in the forearm or hand can share or replace the usual pattern.

Arteries party too. Squeeze your left hand into a fist and then grab your left wrist forcefully with your right hand. Open your left hand partway. The palm is pale because your fist squeezed the blood out and your left hand is preventing its return. Now relax your right thumb while maintaining pressure with the rest of

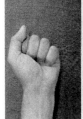
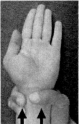
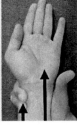

your right hand. How many seconds does it take your palm to turn pink? Do it again; make a fist and grab your wrist. After you open your left hand this time, keep pressure with your right thumb but relax the other fingers. How long did it take your palm to turn pink this time? By releasing the pressure first on one side of your wrist and then the other, you are testing the two major arteries that supply your hand. That is if you have two major arteries. Sometimes one is minor and fills the hand only slowly. Sometimes one is missing. Confusing or interesting?

Double joints seem to be a universal fascination. No, these rubbery people don't have extra hinges. The ones they have are just so loose that they can contort into positions that make the rest of us wince. These people make good gymnasts, who are interesting to watch. Ah, human variation. Appreciate it as hand surgeons do. In one respect, however, our hands cannot vary too far from normal before big problems with activities arise. I am talking about our thumbs.

CIVILIZATION, COURTESY OF THE HUMAN THUMB

Throw a ball, hold a pen, fasten a button. With your thumb in position to do these maneuvers, notice that its contact surface is opposite and facing the contact surfaces of your other fingers. In this position it *opposes* their free movement and allows for throwing strikes, signing papers, and getting dressed. Since the thumb can move in and out of this position, we call it opposable.

Humans rarely give this amazing motion a conscious nod, but combine it with a large brain, let it brew for several hundred thousand years, and voilà, we have civilization. Armed with opposable thumbs, going from rubbing charcoal sticks against cave walls to scribbling on personal digital assistants was only a matter of time. The same is true for hurling rocks and baseballs, scraping and stitching skins into capes, and running a sewing machine. So an opposable thumb is pretty amazing. It is ultimately responsible for everything man-made. Various languages celebrate it in this way. *Shast* in Persian means both "60" and "thumb," signifying that it constitutes 60% of the hand's function. In Turkish, thumb is *bas parmak*—chief finger. And in Latin it is *pollex*, which is derived from *pollere*—to be strong. Isaac Newton marveled, "In the absence of any other proof, the thumb alone would convince me of God's existence."

Because this wonderful digit sticks out somewhat awkwardly and is involved in nearly every manual activity, it is at high risk for injury. Anybody with a severely injured thumb immediately appreciates the complexity of civilization and the difficulties of participation. In case of loss of another finger, three can pretty well do the work of four; but loss of the thumb, with its unique opposability, has devastating consequences. Understanding its importance, hand surgeons work all night if necessary to piece an injured thumb back together. At times a completely amputated thumb can be successfully replanted. Although a replanted thumb is never normal in its sensibility, motion, and strength, it is usually good enough to allow the owner reentry into the human race.

What reconstruction techniques are available when surgeons cannot repair or replant this critical part? Three major methods are available. Call them beg, borrow, and steal.

In the first, the surgeon and patient persuade (beg) the thumb remnant to lengthen. Steel pins and an expandable, external steel frame attach to the ends of the residual bone, which is cut in the middle. Then by turning a little knob, the patient expands the frame in nearly microscopic increments on an hourly basis for several months. The bone and the surrounding muscles, tendons, nerves, and skin hardly know they are being stretched. They just think there is some powerful growing under way, and they rally to keep up. After several months in "the rack" the thumb is nearly back to its normal length. The advantage of this lengthening procedure is that it avoids borrowing or stealing. Its disadvantages are that it does not restore the thumbnail or any missing joints.

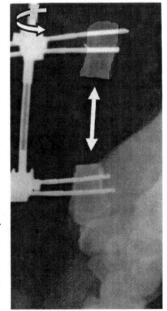

As mentioned earlier, the index, middle, ring, and small fingers work similarly, and losing one of these is not nearly as debilitating as losing a thumb. So what to do when the indispensable thumb is missing and there are four underemployed friends stationed nearby? Hmm. Borrow one? Yes!

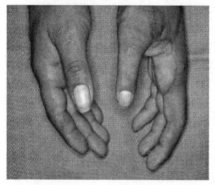

Because of its proximity, the index finger usually gets the call and can be surgically rotated and shortened into the thumb position. This surgery is more complicated than remnant lengthening and leaves a four-digit hand, which is not bad looking. (Cartoon characters all have four-digit hands.) The advantages of borrowing for thumb reconstruction are that the new thumb has a nail and the convalescence is short.

At times, however, other digits from the same hand are missing or the patient has need for a five-digit hand. In either case, there is no finger to borrow. Here the surgeon may resort to theft. The unsuspecting foot is the victim, but nobody ever said that toes were responsible for civilization. Therefore, the crime is merely a misdemeanor. The shape of the big toe is almost identical to the thumb so it is the favored mark, although its theft leaves an ugly crime scene. Stealing the second toe makes for a rather scrawny thumb but leaves a pleasantly contoured foot. Absence of either the first or second toe has minimal effect on the owner's ability to walk and run. Civilization marches on.

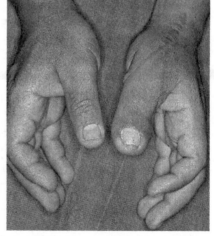

Toe-to-thumb transfer is a 6- to 12-hour operation requiring the finest microsurgical skills. Usually one team of doctors meticulously separates the toe from the foot, carefully protecting the toe's principal artery, vein, nerves, and tendons for later reconnection in the hand. They finally divide the bone, coping with the dilemma of needing to take sufficient length to restore the thumb but leaving as much as possible to maximize foot function. Simultaneously, a second team of surgeons prepares the hand, identifying and mobilizing the ends of all the structures that need connecting to provide stability, nourishment, motion, strength, sensation, and protective covering for the new thumb. The raw bone ends are wired together. Tendons from the toe are sutured to muscles in the forearm. Then using the microscope, a steady hand, and suture so fine that it is nearly invisible to the unaided eye, the surgeon connects the toe artery to a wrist artery and the toe vein to a wrist vein. It is indeed a thrill to unclamp the sutured vessels and watch the toe, now thumb, turn pink. Microsurgically connecting two nerves to restore sensation to the new thumb and suturing the skin closed both in the hand and foot complete the feat.

I think if you ask any hand surgeon what truly lights his fire, he is likely to say thumb reconstruction, be it by begging, borrowing, or stealing. The surgeon's thumbs making a patient's thumb. Just how important is the surgeon's own thumb?

LESS THAN TEN

An article with the above title appeared in *The Journal of Hand Surgery* some years ago. Dr. Paul Brown surveyed nearly 200 surgeons who were missing parts of their hands and reported his findings, which may surprise you.

Dr. Brown was interested in determining how important ten complete fingers are to daily activities. He picked surgeons to survey because of their high level of motivation and their dependence on manual dexterity for their livelihood.

The surgeons' losses ranged from a single fingertip to an entire hand. One sixth of those surveyed were missing major portions of a thumb, and one sixth had loss of more than one finger. Absences were twice as common in dominant as in nondominant hands.

Injury accounted for most of the losses. Power saws and planers were the most frequent offenders, followed by lawn mowers, gears, snow blowers, and farm equipment. A few were from shark and orangutan bites (no kidding). Infection, tumors, and congenital absences accounted for the remaining differences.

Half of those surveyed had sustained their loss before becoming surgeons, including one person who became a surgeon, rather than a pianist, because of his injury. Loss of manual dexterity was an infrequent complaint. Of those who sustained amputations after surgical training, only three had to stop operating.

Twenty-nine surgeons actually found portions of their work easier because of the loss. Their narrower hands allow them to reach into deeper spaces through shorter incisions. The amputation also forced some to become ambidextrous, thereby enhancing their surgical skills.

Some surgeons in the survey use custom-made surgical gloves, but most simply tuck the empty finger(s) inside the palm of the glove. The respondents stated that once they adjusted to their losses and treated them matter-of-factly, then so did their patients. Young children are often the only ones who notice minor amputations, even when present on multiple fingers.

A loss of music-playing proficiency, especially on the piano and stringed instruments, was the most frequently noted change away from work. Nearly all of the surgeons, however, noted no disability in performing self-care and household activities. Some commented that they had given up woodworking or at least were more cautious around power equipment.

Most surgeons stressed that adaptation and incentive were the key factors in resuming function with an injured or deficient hand. Dr. Brown concluded that an individual's motivation is more important for manual activities than ten complete fingers. Nonetheless, ten are nice. Let Roald Dahl help you decide how important yours are.

MAN FROM THE SOUTH

Author Roald Dahl is best known for his children's stories, *James and the Giant Peach* and *Charlie and the Chocolate*

Factory. He also wrote short stories for adults in which characters' lives are changed in dramatic and unexpected ways, surprising both character and reader.

In *Man from the South*, a small old man bets a young sailor that the young man cannot successfully strike his cigarette lighter ten times in a row. Tension mounts quickly when the two finally agree on the stakes for what started as a casual poolside wager. The sailor gets the old man's Cadillac if the lighter works the tenth time. The old man chops off the sailor's little finger if the lighter fails.

Man from the South is an interesting and somewhat macabre read. I am aware of no other work of literature that so succinctly and dramatically weighs a finger's value.

ARTIFICIAL FINGERS

It is natural to be startled when we see a finger with a missing tip, a hand with a missing finger, or an arm with a missing hand. Then surprise may turn to curiosity. How did it happen? I wonder if it hurts. What happens if we have to shake hands, or dance? We suddenly become aware of our hands and their importance to our self-image. Either we acknowledge our good fortune, never see that person again and forget about the encounter, or the person enters our lives. In that case we eventually accept her as a whole individual despite her unique appendage. Sometimes we even get to know her well enough to learn about the origin of her deformity and how it affects her activities and sense of self.

Even if the owners of deficient hands are entirely well adjusted and fully functional, at times they have to withstand stares and winces. Some people with absent fingers use their hands so smoothly that the difference is rarely noticed. Others enhance their self-confidence by hiding their hand. They may do this by leaving the abnormal hand in their lap or adroitly covering it with their normal hand or clothing. Others move through the day with their hands in full sight while we see nothing out of the ordinary.

Perhaps you have encountered a person with an artificial finger or hand and never knew it. Latex rubber substitutions for missing digits can be amazingly lifelike. Of course the substitutes cannot feel or bend, but they can certainly fool the eye. The best ones are custom-tinted to match the owner's skin color. If the junction between living and artificial is covered with a ring or

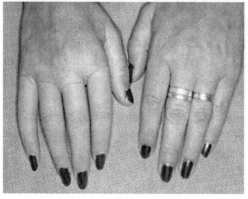

watchband, the substitution can withstand scrutiny without detection. As an additional detail, nails, both artificial and real, can be painted to match each other. In the adjoining figure, the index, middle, ring, and small fingers on the right hand are artificial.

The best prosthetics are expensive. The best single-finger substitutes cost several thousand dollars and partial and whole hand cosmetic replacements cost even more. They are not terribly durable for household activities and may require periodic repair or replacement for tears or staining. Therefore, owners typically reserve their use for when they are out of the house.

Let's see how some people have managed when missing entire hands.

SINGLE-HANDED SUCCESSES

Anyone who has experienced even something as minor as a paper cut or a hangnail knows how annoying it can be to have fewer than ten perfectly functioning fingers. And someone who has had a hand bandaged after an injury or operation knows the frustration of attempting simple two-handed activities such as cutting food, tying shoes, or opening an envelope. Now imagine having only one hand for the rest of your life. Could you get dressed? Type? Drive? Excel in a two-handed world?

Since the invention of gunpowder, the most common war wounds have been the most common way hands and arms are lost. Until the 1940s, amputation was the accepted life-saving treatment for major injuries. Consequently, many military figures of the past achieved success and even fame despite physical handicaps resulting from on-the-job losses.

For instance, Horatio Nelson's right forearm was shattered in a naval battle in 1797 and required amputation—in a pitching boat, no less. Lord Nelson went on, however, to lead the British navy to victory over Napoleon's forces at Trafalgar, empowering Britain's dominion of the seas for an entire century.

There are other examples on this side of the ocean. During the Mexican War, Philip Kearny lost his left hand. Fifteen years later, he distinguished himself as a Union general in the Civil War. A bronze statue of him, absent his hand, marks his grave in Arlington Cemetery.

Captain John Wesley Powell's right elbow was destroyed by gunfire at Shiloh and required amputation two days later. When the Civil War was over, Powell led several expeditions down the then-uncharted Colorado River, riding out Grand Canyon rapids in a chair lashed to the boat's mid-deck. Later he served as director of the U.S. Geological Survey. Lake Powell is named in his honor.

Both Senator Robert Dole from Kansas and Senator Daniel Inouye from Hawaii sustained debilitating upper limb injuries during World War II. One could argue that leadership makes no special demands on the hands, but what about success in manually demanding endeavors?

Consider the one-handed magician, Rene Lavand. This Argentinean prestidigitator has astounded audiences worldwide with his close-up magic. He also lectures to magicians and notes, "It is possible to perform these effects with two hands as well."

Several athletes come to mind. Karli Takash, a Hungarian, won an Olympic gold medal for pistol shooting after switching to his nondominant (and only) hand following an injury.

Jim Abbott, pitcher for the US baseball team in the 1988 Olympics, turned in another gold-medal-level performance. Despite being born with only a thumb on his right hand, Jim learned to deftly remove and replace the glove on his left hand to both field and throw left-handed. In high school he batted .427, quarterbacked his football team, and started as forward in basketball. More recently he distinguished himself with an outstanding major league baseball career.

The North American One-Armed Golfers Association plays an annual tournament against its British counterpart, the Society of One-Armed Golfers. The good players consistently drive 280 yards, and some of them say that pitching and putting with one hand is easier than with two—less to go wrong. Nor does the absence of one arm phase Bahamas fishing guide Marvin Adderley, who fly-fishes single-handedly. He strips out and makes a coil of line behind him and releases it as needed between fingers on his casting hand. When it comes time to reel in a catch, he wedges the rod between his thighs and winds away.

Similar accomplishments, amazing as they may seem, have occurred in music. Paul Wittgenstein was a promising young Austrian concert pianist when World War I exploded across Europe. Paul joined the Austrian army and within a year sustained a right arm wound that required amputation. Following release from concentration camp six months later, he practiced relentlessly to learn to play the piano with his remaining left hand. He collected and performed music that had been written or arranged for one hand, and he also arranged music himself.

Wittgenstein's diligence and one-handed virtuosity inspired such composers as Richard Strauss, Sergey Prokofiev, Maurice Ravel, and Benjamin Britten to write music especially for him. Sony Compact Disc #SK 47188 contains much of this music. You will be hard-pressed, particularly with the Ravel concerto, to recognize the presence of only one hand on the keyboard.

Well, how about drumming? Def Leppard was a rock band in the 1980s. At the height of their international popularity, their drummer, Rick Allen, lost one arm in a car accident. Undeterred, he designed a custom drum set and was back in the band within several months.

Although not as famous as those mentioned so far, another amputee made it easier for others to achieve single-handed success. David Dorrance lost his hand in a sawmill accident in 1909. Today, many such injuries can be successfully repaired using microsurgical techniques. Back then, however, only closure of the amputation stump was possible. Frustrated by the poor function of the "Captain Hook" type of prostheses available, Dorrance devised and patented a system of highly functional and versatile artificial limbs. They look like hooks, but their owners use them to play the piano, fasten buttons, and perform other similarly dexterous activities. (If you want to see somebody using two Dorrance artificial limbs to light a cigarette, rent *The Best Years of Our Lives*. It's a good movie besides—an Academy Award winner. Details in Chapter 10.) The manufacturing company that Dorrance founded continues to lead this important but rarely considered industry nearly 100 years later.

Multiple resources and opportunities are available for people with only one functioning hand and a desire to type or play a musical instrument. The Internet is a great resource for currently available ideas and adaptive devices.

For example, one-handed typing programs are available that center the normal hand over the *g*, *h*, *j*, and *k* keys on a conventional keyboard and show the user how to branch out from there to reach the other keys. Special computer keyboards, called half-QWERTY, call for positioning the healthy hand over the conventional home keys of *a,s,d,* and *f.* The user controls the keys on the left side of the keyboard as usual, but depressing the spacebar converts the left-sided keys into those normally found on the right side of the keyboard. Careful timing of depressing and releasing the space bar generates a space between words.

Various websites also address one-handed musical instruments. Recorders are probably the most easily adaptable by adding keys to cover the holes normally covered by the deficient hand. Each version has its own fingering system.

Brass instruments are played one-handed under normal circumstances, so little modification is required other than a means of supporting and positioning the instrument while playing it with either hand. Video clips on the Internet show an ambitious violin player who straps the bow to his forearm amputation stump and an undaunted cello player who bows with his foot. Less obviously different but far more commonplace are left-handers, myself included.

LEFTIES IN A RIGHTEOUS WORLD

Have you ever wondered about your left-handed friends and relatives? Do we view the world a little differently? Do we march to a different drummer? Are we singled out as being . . . you name it.

For starters, the world's languages certainly are biased against us. In English, left comes from the Anglo-Saxon *lyft*, meaning weak or broken. Left in French is *gauche*, for which the thesaurus rewards us with synonyms such as awkward, blundering, crude, inept, tactless, and unrefined. Thanks a lot, thesaurus. In Italian, *mancino* means deceitful as well as left, in German *linkisch* also means clumsy, in Russian *na levo* means sneaky, and in Spanish *zurdo* also means malicious. Only in Greek do we get a break, where *aristera* also means aristocratic. So to all the weak, crude, deceitful, and malicious aristocrats, let's rise up against world prejudice and demand our rights, er, lefts.

Psychological and linguistic issues aside, southpaws have to cope in a right-handed world. More manufactured goods than you ever imagined are produced to accommodate the 85 to 90 percent of the population that is right-handed. Left-handers have to adapt.

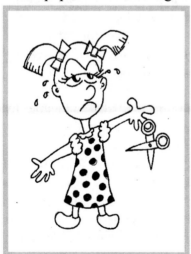

Beginning when we first picked up scissors, lefties sensed that life is unfair. Even an otherwise friendly crayon says *Crayola* upside down when you grasp it in the left hand. Look where the stamps go on envelopes, quite convenient for righties. The lefty wonders, "Am I in the wrong place?" Sure, there are boutiques specializing in left-handed objects (scissors, rulers, coffee mugs), but these are mere novelty items—sinister tokenism.

Where are the cameras with shutter releases and cars with ignition switches for the left hand? Or how about dress shirts with the pocket where it is easily accessible to the left hand, or wristwatches with the stems on the left for dexterous southpaws?

Maybe lefties are supposed to use pocket watches, but if men's trousers have a watch pocket, it is on the right. The pant fly is also designed for right-hand use. The hip pocket with the button to secure one's wallet, however, is on the left. Does this make it easier for southpaws to spend money? Maybe "yes" for foldable money, but not for coins. Just look where the coin slots are on vending machines—situated for right-hand use.

No wonder lefties may be gauche at dinner. Butter knives, serrated knives, dessert forks, and ladles all work great—for the righteous. Even spoons are subtly biased. Yes, hold a spoon in your left hand and turn it over. The writing is upside down. The same goes for pencils and pens

Shoot a shotgun left-handed and the casing ejects into your cheek. Lefties, watch out for power saws of all types. They are not designed for us. Items like these may explain a study done several years ago. It indicated that southpaws do not live as long as the righteous.

Sometimes when I get emotional presenting this diatribe in conversation, righties respond with a smug sense of entitlement, "Well, it's a matter of practicality that manufacturers will do what's right for the vast majority of us." Then why do we have wheelchair ramps at the curbs and braille lettering in elevators? That often brings a look of discovery to their faces and perhaps a little appreciation for what left-handers endure on a daily basis.

"Interesting," you may say, "but how does all this relate to hand surgery?" Well, the score evens out in this area. Because we lefties give our right hands a good workout every day in this right-handed world, a bandage or cast on our left hand still leaves us a dexterous and experienced hand available. Not so for righties, those single-handed successes, who may need to make quick friends with their newly discovered south paw while the north one is out of commission.

It is the same for surgeons. Lefties gradually learn to use right-handed instruments, resulting in ambidextrous skills only dreamed of by the righteous. Furthermore, lefties make terrific first basemen. If you don't understand why, ask a baseball nut.

CHIEF LEFT HAND

Chief Left Hand was a southern Arapaho leader at the time when the white man's migration across the Great Plains challenged the Indians' traditional nomadic ways.

Arapaho means trader, and this tribe relied on peace and free movement to trade with other plains Indians. From such contact with other tribes, Left Hand as a child learned to speak the Cheyenne and Sioux languages. Left Hand's older sister married a white trader, who was impressed with Left Hand's knack for languages and taught him English.

Left Hand's courage and resourcefulness, as well as his command of English, vaulted him to leadership among the southern Arapahos. Opportunistic and mercenary white leaders, however, excluded him whenever possible from treaty negotiations. They could not shade the facts in their favor by muddying the translation when Left Hand was present.

The ultimate affront, however, came in November 1864. Despite the Arapaho's continued conciliatory movements, an overzealous regiment of Colorado territory volunteers swept through Left Hand's encampment. They killed and mutilated over 100 women and children along with the few warriors who were not away hunting. The circumstances of Left Hand's death remain unknown.

What is well established, however, is that following this massacre at Sand Creek, the plains Indians realized that further negotiations with the white settlers were hopeless. This opened up the longest armed conflict in US history—a 25-year guerrilla war that ranged from Texas to Montana and included the well-known Indian payback to General Custer.

Ironically, the southern Arapaho did not join the war. They wandered the southern plains and never returned to Colorado. Ultimately, white men recognized Left Hand's attributes. His English name became attached to Left Hand Canyon just north of Boulder, Colorado, and his Arapaho name, Niwot, was given to a nearby town, which was the site of his village, and to a mountain among the Indian Peaks of the Rockies.

GO LEFT, YOUNG MAN

To get to Left Hand, West Virginia, you can either take the land route or the water route. To best understand Left Hand, get a paddle and some waders. Head northeast out of Charleston, West Virginia, up the Elk River. One of its major tributaries is Big Sandy Creek. Go that way. You will come 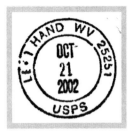 to a branch on the port side. Don't go there. That's Little Left Hand Run. Farther up and also on the left is another branch. Take it. You're probably wading by now. In a few miles you will see a scattering of houses, barns, and garden patches alongside Left Hand Run. Welcome to Left Hand. Just upstream is Looneyville. Go figure.

WHERE DID "SOUTHPAW" COME FROM?

The expression "southpaw" to describe a left-handed person originates from Chicago sportswriters in the 1890s, when all the games were played during the day. Baseball diamonds were oriented so that home plate was the southwest corner of the square. That way, the batters looked away from the sun during the late afternoon. For a left-handed pitcher or first baseman facing home plate, his ungloved, left hand was his south paw.

Up to this point, we have considered the hand through time and through life and its role at work, even when deficient. Let's look at the hand when it is just having fun.

CHAPTER

5

Athletic and Playful

HANDS

I MAGINE WALKING 16 MILES IN A DAY. THEN THINK ABOUT doing that every day for two months. That would get you from Denver to St. Louis, from New York to Atlanta, or from Seattle to San Francisco. In 1900 Austrian Johann Hurlinger walked that distance (870 miles) from Paris to Vienna—on his hands Yes, he made a lasting name for himself, but the view couldn't have been that great from two feet off the ground and upside down. This chapter explores some of the other stresses the hand absorbs in the name of recreation.

SHOULDER 101

The hand's marvelous versatility comes in part from its ability to move widely in space. For instance, it can touch the body's entire surface and also move away from the torso in all directions. Athletic endeavors, gymnastics, and throwing sports, for example, highlight this ability for the hand to move widely and at times also quickly and forcefully. To a great extent, this spatial adaptability comes from the shoulder, which is not a single joint, but three or four, depending on how you count.

The shoulder starts where the collarbone attaches to the breastbone just below the throat. This is the shoulder's only bony connection with the torso, which accounts in part for the shoulder's great mobility. The collarbone serves as a strut between the torso and the shoulder blade and allows the shoulder blade to move widely yet securely on the chest wall, such as with shoulder

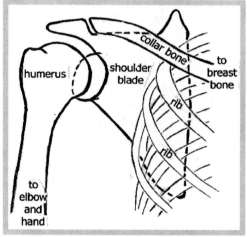

shrugging. Next the round end of the upper arm bone, the humerus, forms a shallow ball-and-socket joint with the shoulder blade. These three real joints and the motion between the shoulder blade and the chest wall combine to make the shoulder the most mobile of any linkage in the body.

Strong yet flexible ligaments securely link the breastbone, collarbone, shoulder blade, and humerus together. Then an amazing array of muscles connects the shoulder bones to one another and to the skull, spine, ribs, pelvis, and forearm to get the hand moving. That is the good news.

The bad news is that this highly mobile, intricate system is a little fragile. The shoulder is especially susceptible to broken bones, displaced and worn out joints, irritated tendons, and stiffened ligaments. Not much has to be wrong in any of these categories before hand mobility becomes restricted. Hence, a sore shoulder can profoundly affect recreational activities such as golf, tennis, weight lifting, and throwing.

And alas, come Monday morning, it can limit work activities in situations where the hand has to be in a wide variety of positions--building trades, for instance. Even for sedentary individuals, a stiff, painful shoulder makes dressing and sleeping difficult. It is worse for elderly people, especially if they have limited flexibility and strength in other joints. A bad shoulder may even preclude independent living.

Shoulders do not get the respect they deserve. True, a shoulder cannot dunk basketballs or tee up a golf ball, but without a good shoulder, the hand's virtuosity is limited. Some hand surgeons include the shoulder in their domain of expertise; others do not. It is wise to ask before you make an appointment. Hand surgeons who do not treat shoulders can certainly empathize with your problem and direct you to specialty care. When the shoulder and elbow are feeling fine, what can they do with a baseball?

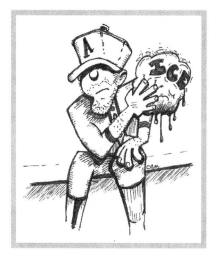

THE SPIN ON BASEBALL

A fastball pitch in baseball speeds toward the plate with a backspin on it. A curve has a sidespin. The stitched, slightly raised seams on the spinning baseball react with the air rushing by at 70 to 100 miles per hour, making the ball fight gravity longer in the case of a fastball or veer off to the side in the case of a curve. A knuckle ball has no spin on it and acts erratically depending on which seam happens to catch the most air.

Pitching rosin helps a pitcher keep his fingertips dry and tacky even during hot humid weather. This allows him a better grip on the ball for inducing a sidespin and producing a wicked curve. Conversely, substances like saliva or petroleum jelly make the tips of the index and middle fingers slippery—resulting in a pitch with the speed and motion of a fastball but with less backspin. To the batter it looks like a fastball, but it sinks faster. Because it is so difficult to hit, the spit ball is against the rules.

THE WIDE WORLD OF SPORTS INJURIES

It is one thing to endure a little tendonitis around the shoulder or elbow or an occasional sprained finger because of baseball, volleyball, or basketball, but can you imagine routinely risking a broken wrist or an amputated thumb for the sake of sport?

Certain athletic activities expose the hands to extreme forces and dangers that are well known to hand surgeons and to some of the sports' participants. You too might want to familiarize yourself with these risks before trading in your golf clubs for a spot on the bowling or rodeo circuit, especially if you have other uses for your hands, a day job for instance.

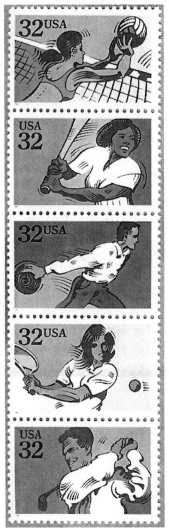

Obviously sports where one throws one's opponent to the ground has bodily implications for the to-be-thrown, but there are also implications for the thrower, especially if the to-be-thrown resists and runs away. Known to hand surgeons as rugger jersey finger, this tendon problem occurs when the thrower grabs for the jersey of the departing rugby or football player. It also happens if a player gets his finger caught in a basketball net. A forceful and sudden straightening out of the hooked finger can detach one of the fist-making tendons from its bony attachment, leaving the thrower with an inability to curl into the palm the joint closest to the fingernail. The ring finger is the usual victim, and if the tendon is not surgically reattached in its normal location within a few days after injury, the thrower will have a lifetime memento of the event. So maybe you want to think about a less violent sport.

How about bowling? Is it safe provided you don't drop the ball on your toes? Not completely. The risk here is bowler's thumb, which is numbness on the thumb's contact surface. The loss of sensation makes the handling of small objects, like buttons, paper clips, and earrings, difficult if not impossible. The problem stems from the edge of the bowling ball's thumbhole repeatedly pressing hard into the nerve that supplies sensation to the thumb's contact surface. Think of it as hitting your funny bone every time you pick up a bowling ball. The irritation results in scarring and thickening of the nerve with a loss of its ability to conduct electrical messages. Treatment is not particularly helpful, so this is an injury to avoid or catch early. Help includes redrilling of the ball's thumbhole and then inserting the thumb only part way to minimize pressure on this important, match-stick-diameter nerve.

Want something a little more thrilling than bowling? Something outdoors but with less body contact than football? How about dirt bike racing? Dress up in leather, spew mud on your opponents, soar over jumps, and hang on for dear life. Not only do your hands keep you from flying away, they also work the throttle, clutch, and brake. This continuous forceful gripping causes what the insiders call "arm pump." The forearm turns hard and painful, and the grip goes to mush. The immediate options are to stop or crash. Means of avoiding arm pump include holding on with your knees, conditioning the forearm muscles, and modifying the bike in two ways, first to dampen vibrations and second to soften the clutch action. Some riders have forearm surgery to release the thin, unyielding covering over the muscles. The idea is to let the muscles swell without constriction and pain. This is not completely effective. Perhaps diving can provide the needed thrill without the ache.

Imagine this. Jump off a platform three stories tall. Do a few flips and spins. Then if you decide to go into the water head first, quickly get your hands in front of you, otherwise the impact of the water will break your neck and collarbone. Remember, this is recreation.

Divers from the 10-meter (about 33 feet) platform are moving 30-35 miles an hour when they hit the water. They have two different techniques for saving their necks and leaving a minimal splash. Try it—the hand position, not the dive. Make a fist with one hand with your thumb sticking out. Now grab that thumb with your other hand and make a fist around it. Put your hands overhead and imagine punching a hole in the water and scoring a 9. The newer and more often used technique makes a bigger hole, which slows the body faster and awards the diver with only a tiny ripple and a possible 10. This entails hitting the water with your open palm supported from behind with your other open palm.

To get to the Olympics, plan on diving 240 times per week and having chronic pain in your wrists. Torn tendons, torn ligaments, and broken wrist bones go with the territory. Use a Velcro hook and loop wrist wrap during training and do as much of your practice as possible from lesser heights and on a trampoline. Before you decide to give up diving and take up steer roping, however, consider this.

Instruction manuals for rodeo riders contain such recommendations as: "Keep your thumb up during the dally. If your thumb is down, it can get caught between the rope and the saddle horn and be cut off." Every year, hand surgeons take care of some cowboys who did not heed this advice. What happens?

Once the steer is lassoed, the rider quickly wraps his end of the rope around the saddle horn (the dally) to keep the rope from running through his hands as the steer veers off. If the thumb is not kept out of the way, it gets crushed between the suddenly tightening coils of rope and the saddle horn. Yes, this is a nasty injury and only sometimes can a surgeon successfully reattach an amputated thumb. Remarkably, some riders prefer not to have a replantation even attempted, saying that their thumbless buddies dally better than ever! Tennis anyone? No, that has problems that I'll tell you about in Chapter 6 along with baseball injuries. How about skiing, rock climbing, skating, and boxing?

SKIER'S THUMB

For grasping, pinching, and manipulation of various-sized objects, our thumbs are indispensable. Imagine, for example, trying to turn a key or fasten a button without using your thumb. Since the thumb is shorter, stronger, and uniquely positioned in comparison to the other digits, it can resist their motions and forces. To do its work, however, the thumb requires a combination of mobility *and* stability. Necessary mobility may be lacking whenever the joints are stiff from injury or arthritis. Stability depends on one key ligament.

This ligament spans the thumb's middle joint on the index-finger side. It resists the other fingers' efforts to push the thumb away from the palm during pinching and gripping activities. When it is healthy, we never give this tough, flexible, ½ inch long by ¼ inch wide ligament any thought. When it is injured, however, the thumb is practically useless. Now the thumb floats aimlessly away from the palm rather than opposing the remaining digits. Forceful grasping and pinching are impossible.

Almost everyone is familiar with ankle sprains, when ligaments are stretched or torn and the foot is suddenly forced into an unnatural position. The same thing can happen to the thumb if it is violently forced away from the palm. For example, in automobile accidents the thumb may get caught across the steering wheel, and in basketball the thumb may be sprained against another player or a flying ball.

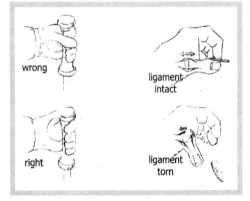

Thumb ligament injuries are particularly common during ski season. A fall, even while standing still, can force the ski pole handle against the thumb, thus tearing this ligament. The style of the pole handle, with or without a strap, seems to make no difference.

Of course, for skiers, the best prevention is not to fall. The next best and more practical advice is to ski with your thumbs on top of the poles rather than around them. From this position, the handle cannot wedge between your thumb and palm during a fall.

Whether from skiing or from other causes, thumb ligament injuries deserve special attention. If the ligament is just slightly stretched, wearing a protective cast or splint for a month or so promotes the necessary healing. If the ligament is completely torn and displaced, only a surgical procedure can restore it. When such an injury receives treatment within several weeks of occurrence, the ends of the torn ligament can simply be reattached. Otherwise, a ligament reconstruction—borrowing a relatively unimportant tendon from elsewhere in the body and lacing it through holes in the bone like a shoestring--can restore the thumb's former and critical stability. Either surgical repair or reconstruction probably won't get you back on the slopes the same season, but there is always rock climbing when the weather warms up.

A FLY ON THE WALL

Some years back, I took care of a rock climber with a broken finger, a scalp laceration, and a minor skull fracture. She was clinging, several thousand feet off the ground, to a sheer rock face in Yosemite when a climber above her dislodged some stones. She protected her head with her hand, and the crush injury to her finger likely saved her life. This was a night climb, so she had to hold on until morning for a helicopter rescue. When the fracture healed and with some stiffness in one digital joint, she went back to climbing with her previous ferocity.

This sounds fanatical to most of us, but when you talk to climbers, this story is just another day on the rock. They speak of self-reliance, stamina, choreography, conditioning, challenge, focus. To scale rock faces that appear unblemished, these intrepid athletes capitalize on minor irregularities in the stone for foot and hand holds. Ledges as narrow as an eighth of an inch and cracks and holes big enough for only a single finger offer potential for human attachment. Then it is merely a matter of finding a sequence of "holds" spaced within reach and figuring out how to move among them.

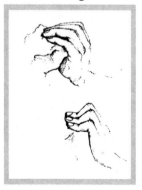

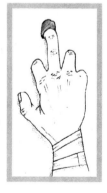

Several different grips are standard. The *open grip* is used on large handholds such as big knobs and edges. The *cling grip* is used on smaller edges. One or two fingers may be inserted into a small hole forming the *pocket grip.*

Cracks in the rock offer several other options. There may be small ledges within the crack to allow gripping. Otherwise, the climber can insert finger, fist, or foot, twist the part until it locks against the unyielding stone, and move upward. Gloves are shunned because they diminish the sense of touch and reduce the security of handholds. Skin abrasions and heavy calluses are commonplace as are sprained joints and inflamed tendons.

Upper body conditioning is critical. Conventional weight training is just a beginning. Then comes cling-grip chin-ups on door moldings, first grasping with eight fingertips and aiming toward the goal of two-finger pull-ups or even a one-finger pull-up. Contrasted with most other human endeavors, the thumbs are relatively unimportant in rock climbing.

The sport is growing in popularity. Many gyms, even home gyms, now include climbing walls where various-sized knobs, ledges, and pockets are bolted to vertical and even overhanging surfaces to simulate natural rock formations. In the flatlands where rock formations are sparse, climbing clubs train inside empty grain elevators.

So the next time you see a fly walking up a smooth wall, appreciate that human hands allow similar maneuvers. It is just that we can't buzz away—at least without a helicopter.

AVOIDING SKATING INJURIES

Roller skating has taken on new popularity with the development of in-line skates. Speeds in excess of 25 mph are possible, but injuries also occur while skaters are standing still. Many injuries that affect the hand, wrist, and elbow are preventable if the following measures are taken:

- Perform stretching exercises before skating.
- Wear wrist, elbow, and knee protectors and a helmet.
- Put on protective gear before putting on skates.
- Learn how to stop safely on flat and gently inclined surfaces before getting fancy.

Just as wrist guards provide some protection while skating, specialized gloves used for cycling, hockey, and handball afford some safety. In other sports such as baseball and golf, gloves facilitate the function of the hand. Do boxers use gloves to protect their hands, to facilitate their effectiveness, or to protect their adversary?

BRAWLERS AND BOXERS

Hands are marvelous instruments and can express love in many ways. They have their dark side, however, because they can also express anger and violence. These negative strokes range from finger pointing to fist shaking, fist pounding, slaps, and slugs. One of the most common fractures in the hand comes from fisticuffs, and learning how to avoid the injury also reveals something interesting about how bones work. So if you are interested for either reason, read on.

Despite its hard, rock-like nature, bone is alive. It grows and it can mend itself. Amazingly, it responds to the stresses it receives by getting tougher, just like frequent gardening without gloves produces calluses. The bones in an avid tennis player's dominant forearm, for instance, become measurably thicker and stronger than on the side not subjected to the repeated stresses. If she stops playing for a few months, the bones in both forearms are identically dense and strong. Another example is the metacarpal bones in the hand—those five bones inside the palm. We subject our metacarpals to various stresses during gripping and lifting activities and they stay in shape to withstand the pressures generated by these activities. But do something they haven't prepared for, like fisting a wall, and they break.

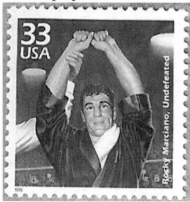

Here is where bone biology separates the barroom brawler from the experienced bare-fisted boxer. The brawler is usually a roundhouse swinger, and his fist flies in a curve on the end of a pendulum. The little finger's metacarpal is the first thing that encounters anything hard. The metacarpal has no experience in resisting such bending forces. It breaks. (The thugs in the movies use brass knuckles, which transfer the impact from the closed fist to the palm, which supposedly is stronger.) The boxer, by contrast, usually punches as if his fist is on the end of a piston, hitting straight on. The metacarpal is stronger at withstanding these end-on forces than the bending forces sustained by the brawler's hand. The boxer has also conditioned his bones over months of repeated impacts in practice. The boxer's metacarpals have gotten stronger just like the tennis player's forearm bones, so they are far more likely to withstand the occasional roundhouse swing without breaking.

The bad news for boxers is that the repeated impacts on the joints between the metacarpals and the wrist bones lead to early arthritis, which may be career ending. The good news for brawlers is that their fractures usually heal completely after three to four weeks in a cast. If they don't go to anger management class, however, they may do it again. Here is a story that hand surgeons hear from time to time. "I was angry and punched through the wall board. I've done it a hundred times. This time I must have hit a stud."

For those who are interested in a little hand-to-hand combat but disdain the idea of broken noses, consider arm wrestling. In recent years this traditional kitchen table and tavern pastime has become a full-fledged sport with official rules, competitions, and international rankings. Technique is important. If good, it can at times trump brute strength. If bad, that bruiser holding your hand can break your arm.

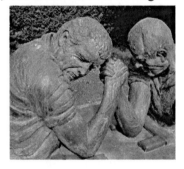

A LIFETIME OF AMUSEMENT

Many of us prefer less strenuous and less risky sports. For instance, take cat's cradle—weaving a loop of string stretched around opposing fingers into various patterns. This simple diversion for self and others seems timeless. The same goes for finger and hand puppets. Juggling too, but this requires a higher commitment to hand-eye coordination. Depending on your age, you may recall playing jacks, marbles, mumblety-peg, Atari, or Nintendo. Do you also remember bending your index around the tip of your thumb and inking adjoining surfaces to make an amusing and heavy-lipped friend? In every instance our hands are playthings, but the hand needs an accessory, sometimes quite simple, to get in the game. What about amusements where the hands alone suffice?

For me, hand games started with patty-cake. If my parents played it to convince me to be a baker, it didn't work. I don't remember which came next, church and steeple or itsy bitsy spider. Together, they provided minutes of early childhood entertainment but not to any sustained interest in architecture or arachnology. When I was about six somebody told me I could see a sausage between the tips of my straight and touching index fingers if I brought them near the bridge of my nose. I didn't get it at first because I was looking for a sausage patty rather than a link. Maybe with that expansive line of thought I was destined to be a butcher, but about that time a cool family friend showed me the momentarily-detached-thumb trick. Perhaps that kindled my interest in hand surgery.

By fifth grade, my rowdy buddies and I wrestled--thumb wrestling in confined spaces and Indian wrestling if the breakables were at least a foot away. Then came hot hands. Previously, hand games were simple poetry or brute strength, but hot hands required speed, agility, and concentration. My hands would stay red for days when I lost.

Next came the cerebral rush with winning a few rounds of rock, paper, scissors. I never developed a strategy for sustained victory and lost interest. I slowly wandered away from my buddies toward the less-structured and remarkably pleasant pastime of holding hands. Eventually this led to being the patty-caker rather than the patty-cakee, and the cycle started again. I hope to have a third round of patty caking, this time with grandchildren, before twiddling my thumbs into the sunset with maybe an occasional round of church and steeple if nobody is watching.

SHADOW FIGURES

As long as I am reminiscing about childhood games, let's go way back. It was probably only several minutes after one of my caveman ancestors brought the first burning branch home that some smarty nephew began using the flickering light to cast shadows of his hands on the wall. Neat stuff for a few more minutes, until the cave got so smoky that everybody ran out into the cold. As more advanced forms of lighting came along, shadow figures became more sophisticated as well. Books from a century ago were filled with illustrations of contorted hand postures used for making a whole menagerie of silhouettes from alligators to wombats. It seems to be a lost art.

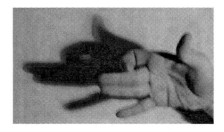

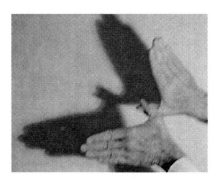

6

HANDS

Through the Year

T RUE OR FALSE:

1. Frostbite occurs more commonly in Baltimore than in Minneapolis.

2. Heat works better than ice for week-old sprains.

3. Most people with tennis elbow have not touched a racket in years.

4. Breaking pieces of thawing food apart with a knife is a bad idea.

The answers to these questions may not be intuitive, but they are important for maintaining hands in top condition. As the seasons change, so do the perils that afflict hands. Here is a month-by-month account of what can happen to hands through the year and information on maintenance and repair. (All four of the above statements are true, so unless you got them all right, read on.)

JANUARY: NEW HANDS FOR THE NEW YEAR

New Year's babies in diapers and party hats remind us that January begins a new life cycle. The Roman god Janus gives the month its name. He is identified with all beginnings since he had two faces—one looking forward, one looking backward.

Rare indeed are babies born with two faces. More common than you might think, however, are babies born with unusual hands. What can these children look forward to in their new year?

The most amazing event of all is that from a single, microscopic, fertilized cell, most of us develop normally. When differences in hand formation do occur, some are genetically transmitted and tend to run in families. Generally, however, the cause is subtle and eludes identification.

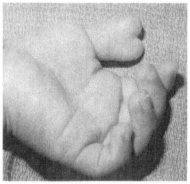

Extra fingers in various forms are the most common hand differences seen in newborns. Pediatricians and obstetricians in the newborn nursery routinely remove the relatively common, incompletely formed nubbins that may attach to the small finger's base. Major duplications require the thoughtful, meticulous attention of a hand surgeon to construct the best possible hand for both function and appearance.

Webbed fingers are also common. Partial webs are exceedingly common between toes, especially the second and third

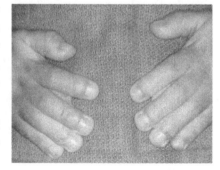

ones. Webbed toes are generally inconsequential, whereas webbed fingers greatly impair spread-finger activities, such as playing chords on the piano and grasping large objects. Also, when a shorter finger is tethered to a longer one, such as when the thumb is webbed to the index, the longer one gets pulled sideways because it grows faster. So separating them improves function and maintains alignment. As is the case for extra fingers, the surgery for webbed fingers is far more complex than just splitting the skin. In addition to the fingers sharing skin, they may also be sharing crucial arteries and nerves and even bone, in which case the surgeon meticulously teases these tissues apart. For complete coverage, skin grafts, usually taken from the groin area, are almost always necessary. Surgeons generally wait until the child is one to two years old before separating the webs. It is easier then to see underlying nerves and arteries and to sew in the tiny skin grafts.

The third large category of congenital hand problems is missing parts. The presence of an incompletely formed thumb renders an otherwise well-formed hand almost useless. In this instance, removal of the inadequate thumb and con-struction of a new one using the index finger is the time-honored choice.

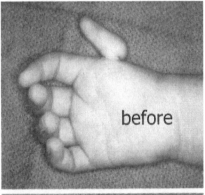

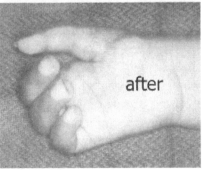

Surgery is less effective at treating more extensive ab-sences, and use of a partial or complete artificial hand is the best decision for some chil-dren. Microsurgical transfer of toes can replace some missing parts. The anticipated im-provement of hand function must outweigh the effects of narrowing and deforming the foot. To avoid the problems of rejection, the toe(s) must come from the patient's own foot for now.

Looking backward, we still do not understand why most of these abnormalities occur, but there are effective surgical techniques for dealing with many of them. Looking forward to a

January some years from now, cadaver transplants and even limb regeneration, both to be discussed in Chapter 11, will offer even better solutions.

The website www.limbdifferences.org is an excellent online resource for families and friends of children with unusually formed hands.

FEBRUARY: FROSTBITE

Frostbite describes freezing of body parts. First the skin gets cold and turns white. As the nearby nerves shut down, the part gets tingly, then numb. If complete freezing occurs, ice crystals form inside of the cells and kill them. Toes, noses, and fingertips are particularly vulnerable because they are at the end of the receiving line for warm blood from the body's toasty interior. When there is not enough warm blood to go around, the brain constricts the skin circulation to save the hot stuff for itself and other internal organs that it considers crucial. People have tried overriding this life-sustaining reflex by drinking alcohol, which will in the short run dilate the skin's blood vessels and give the fingers and toes a warm blush. The body, however, is losing heat faster than it is making it, therefore more blood to the digits leads to general body cooling, which risks hypothermia and death. So in the case of impending frostbite, think of alcohol as embalming fluid rather than antifreeze.

The people most vulnerable to frostbite are those who unexpectedly become exposed to cold and have inadequate protection. For example, schoolchildren may leave home in the morning dressed appropriately for a mild winter day. If a storm develops, the temperature may drop suddenly and the children may be unaware of the danger and poorly protect themselves for the trip home. This would more likely occur in a central band across the United States rather than in areas that are consistently cold or warm. But in mountain or desert areas at any latitude, a day hiker may get lost and be unprepared for the sudden drop in temperature at nightfall.

Skiers, mountain climbers, snowmobilers, and other outdoor enthusiasts should regularly check each other for waxy gray noses, cheeks, and fingertips. This indicates that blood is no longer reaching the skin and that immediate care is necessary.

Where the recommendation to rub the freezing part with snow came from, I do not know, but it is a bad one. This would only add a mechanical irritation to the thermal injury. Rapid rewarming of the cold or frozen parts by immersing the affected hands and feet in 104°F water is the mainstay of treatment. This is best done in an emergency room where generalized hypothermia and dehydration can be treated simultaneously.

Anybody who has had his or her toes go numb from cold knows that the rewarming process can be uncomfortable. Water at 104°F is about as hot as one can stand under normal conditions, so another benefit of thawing frozen parts in the emergency room rather than elsewhere is the availability of painkillers. The process can spare cells not yet completely frozen. They will likely respond by forming blisters, and it usually takes weeks before it becomes obvious how much tissue damage is permanent. Digital amputations are, sadly, permanent reminders of winter plans gone awry. Don't forget your mittens. And don't lose them!

MARCH: FIRE OR ICE?

March weather can be unpredictable. People can slip on the tennis court one day and on an icy parking lot the next. With sprains and strains, the question always arises, "Should I put ice or heat on it, Doctor?"

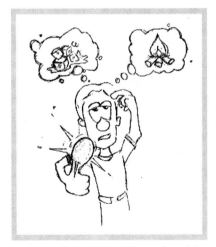

First off, there is very little solid science supporting any thermal treatment. There are certainly millions of muscle and joint problems that have gotten well without any special attention from hot packs or ice bags. Heating or cooling the skin by no means guarantees a thermal change in the deeper structures. Since everybody seems to have an opinion, however, let's make ours as scientific as possible.

The well-known and measurable effects of warmth include muscle relaxation, decreased joint stiffness, increased blood flow, increased flexibility of tissues, and pain relief. The recognized benefits of cold are reduced muscle tone and spasm, increased muscle strength and endurance, increased pain threshold, and reduced bleeding.

Any injury to a muscle or joint goes through several phases of recovery. A sudden injury causes bleeding into torn tissues. A more chronic, repetitive injury may just allow oozing of noxious chemicals from the damaged cells. Either way, the leakage causes swelling and pain. The leakage also awakens reparative cells locally and calls in other healing cells from a distance. These early phases of healing happen over a matter of days.

More slowly, specialized clean-up cells digest and haul away damaged tissues and old blood. New capillaries grow into the area bringing needed oxygen and other nutrients, especially to the cells producing scar tissue. Think of scar tissue as glue. As the glue sets, mending ensues, but structures that previously glided past each other may become stuck to each other. These steps occur over weeks. The extra capillaries finally disappear, and that bright red appearance of the skin that is characteristic of a recent injury abates.

Remarkably, the whole repair process is not complete for roughly six months. How do we intelligently use hot and cold to facilitate the healing and ease the pain?

Apply cold early to reduce bleeding, swelling, pain, and muscle spasm. A simple bag of ice is the best method of delivery. Also, elevation helps immensely. Don't take my word for it, I will show you. While sitting, put your hand in your lap and look at the veins on the back of your hand. They are probably raising the skin a little. Now hold your hand at eye level, and watch those veins flatten out. Raising the injured part reduces its blood pressure, which minimizes fluid leakage, swelling, and painful stretching. Lying down, the sore hand should be up on pillows. The best place for an injured hand while you are walking or standing is on top of your opposite shoulder if not on top of your head. (That's what heads are for, isn't it?) Slings may have a use in shoulder and elbow rehabilitation and for wounded-patriot costumes, but they are generally detrimental for hand and wrist injuries. They let the hand fill up with blood, which makes it hurt. Slings make the shoulder stiff and the neck ache. Bad, bad, bad, but I digress.

After several days, swelling has maxed out. At this point heat, in the form of warm water soaks, a microwavable pack, or an electric heating pad, enhances the circulation to bring needed healing elements to the site and to carry away toxic byproducts. And even later, heat helps recover joint mobility by softening stiff tissues and by relaxing tight muscles. One thing for sure, Epsom salt in the water does not help heal bruises and sprains. Its only potential benefit would be for cleaning up abrasions and scratches.

So for the first several days after a sudden sprain, bruise, or jam, as much ice, rest, and elevation as possible will minimize swelling and pain. The edema and discomfort usually peak at two to four days, then it is time to change to heat. This is practically applied three to four times daily during 10-minute sessions. A stretching program is often included.

For chronic injuries like tennis elbow, the science really gets shaky, but you might try warming up the sore area before strenuous activity, icing it down immediately afterward and using heat on the intervening days of light activity. Of course, the Finns find it refreshing to go back and forth several times in rapid succession from sauna to icy lake water. So try it all and then do what feels good.

THE MYSTIQUE OF EPSOM SALT

A mineral spring was discovered in Epsom, England, about 400 years ago and became the site of a trendy spa. The principal mineral in the water there, magnesium sulfate, remains well known. First used as a laxative, Epsom salt has several useful and many supposedly beneficial properties. When used as a soak or applied to a wet bandage, it draws fluid out of an open wound and is useful for drying up weeping abrasions and scratches.

Epsom salt is also an elixir for growing champion tomatoes and sweet oranges, and you can frost a window by painting it with Epsom salt dissolved in stale beer.

Other uses abound but are without scientific support. Since the outer layer of our skin is both waterproof and magnesium sulfate proof, the soothing effects of a mineral bath are due to the warm water, not the salt. If the skin feels smoother afterward, it is probably due to a fine frosting of salt crystals on the surface. Epsom salt is said to improve the body and remove oil from hair, reduce the effects of autism, and repel raccoons. So if any of these are problems while you are soaking an ailing joint in warm water, have some Epsom salt handy; otherwise save it for scabs and scratches.

APRIL: TAKE ME OUT OF THE BALL GAME

"Sorry 'bout that pop-up, Coach. I lost it in the sun. Look what it did to my finger. It doesn't hurt much, but I can't straighten the last joint."

"That's going to take you out of the line-up for six weeks, Pepper. Why didn't you reach for the ball with your gloved hand or just let it hit you on the head?"

"Come on, give me a break. It's the first game of the year. I'm a little rusty. Haven't you ever hurt any fingers?"

"Yeah, a bunch of times. Why do you think I'm here coaching? Baseball, basketball, football, volleyball—all of 'em can be

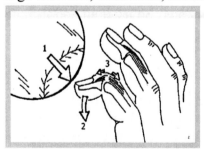 pretty tough on fingers. If the player misjudges even slightly, the ball can send the finger in a direction it's not supposed to go. Better get your ring off right now, before the finger swells and the ring cuts off the circulation."

"Good idea. Thanks. So what exactly happened to me—why does the finger droop? And can I have that stick when you finish your Popsicle?"

"The ball hit your fingertip and bent the joint down so fast it tore the tendon there at the base of the nail. So now the tendon can't lift the joint out of its bent position. I call it baseball finger, others say mallet finger. Anytime the finger is suddenly bent, even jamming it while tucking in the bedspread or forcefully pushing off socks, pow, there it. . . . Hey, get away from my Popsicle. The doctor will fit you with a real splint. The best is a custom-molded plastic splint that holds the joint straight for six weeks or so. The tendon will heal back to its normal length, and like magic, you'll be back on the field dropping flies again."

"Very funny. Say, since you're so smart, look at my other hand. Over a month ago my Great Dane lunged on her leash, which was wrapped around my ring finger. The middle joint's still swollen and stiff, especially in the morning."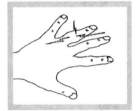

"Yep, leashes—they're a good way to sprain fingers. Horse reins, same thing. You should hold them loosely between you fingers but not wrap them around. Otherwise your finger may veer off while you stay put. Like baseball and basketball injuries, these sprains and dislocations generally don't break the bones but can lead to permanently unstable or stiff fingers if neglected. I'm living proof—see?"

"Hey, show me that again. Fingers aren't supposed to bend that way."

"Yeah, I know. Now. After the flexible tissues around these small finger joints get torn, the rehab's a tricky balance between rest and motion. Too much coddling makes 'em stiff, too much motion makes 'em wobbly. Unfortunately, I treated these injuries myself, and now all I can do is ride the bench."

"Aw, stop it. You're a great coach. You know everything about sports and jammed fingers. And your hands are safe here in the dugout. Let me be your assistant while my finger's healing."

MAY: MOTHER'S HANDS

On Mother's Day, we celebrate women's triumph over the well known perils of child rearing—frazzled nerves, chronic exhaustion, and eternal carpool. But the celebration should extend to mothers' confrontation of lesser known perils as well, including two hand conditions.

One is a nerve entrapment, the other a tendon irritation. The first is carpal tunnel syndrome, where a pinched nerve at the wrist causes numbness and tingling in the fingers. This often occurs during pregnancy. Of course, you don't have to be pregnant to get carpal tunnel syndrome. This common condition also results from faulty wrist position during keyboard activities or from sleeping with your hands curled under your chin. And sometimes it occurs for no reason at all.

Pregnancy and the associated fluid retention in the last several months can deliver the median nerve an extra whammy. The nerve runs through a rigid bony tunnel at the wrist, the carpal canal, and the extra fluid squeezes on the nerve. This causes a pins-and-needles sensation in the fingers, especially at night. If the pressure worsens, constant numbness and burning sensations ensue, which only exacerbate sleepless nights and bloated days.

Treatment during this time includes using a wrist splint to prevent further compression of the nerve and possibly injecting cortisone into the tunnel to reduce swelling in the nerve's vicinity. Symptoms generally begin going away within days after delivery, and carpal tunnel release for pregnancy-related carpal tunnel syndrome is rarely needed.

The other condition, tendonitis at the wrist, comes later, usually when the baby is eight to nine months old. Mom's repetitive cradling and lifting of the baby takes a toll on two tendons at the thumb's base, especially as baby is bulking up but not yet walking. Imagine putting your hands under an infant's arms to lift her up. Now imagine doing it constantly against increasing resistance. The friction, swelling, and inflammation cause sharp pain with any wrist or thumb motion. Finally, imagine trying to get through the day without using your wrists or thumbs while dealing with dirty diapers, frazzled nerves, and chronic exhaustion. Holding Junior for breast-feeding adds further unaccustomed and irritating forces on these tendons.

This type of tendonitis is named after a Swiss doctor, Fritz de Quervain, who described it over 100 years ago. He reported the condition in a washerwoman who was wringing out wet clothes all day long. The same mechanical irritation can cause deQuervain's tendonitis in mothers with adopted babies, even grandmothers, but fathers only rarely, probably because men seem to have fewer opportunities to lift babies and wring laundry.

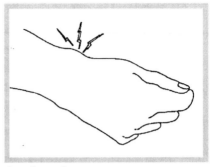

Modern treatment includes a cortisone injection placed around the inflamed tendons. This helps the tendons heal while buying time until Junior is walking and not needing to be picked up as often. But of course by then carpooling is on the horizon.

JUNE: ANIMAL BITES

Ah, summertime. Long idyllic days, less clothing, back to nature. This serenity can be disturbed, however, if some natural beauty sinks its fangs into your hand.

Many bites occur when we startle, corner, or otherwise threaten an animal on its home turf and it acts instinctively to protect itself. So let creatures know your peaceful intentions. For example, don't threaten a snarling dog by making prolonged eye contact. Remain still until the dog loses interest, then back away slowly. Don't run, because it is the dog's natural instinct to chase and catch prey. Be particularly wary around sick, injured, feeding, or nursing animals, who have a heightened sense of self.

Practicing such animal psychology obviously has its limits, however, because Americans report over two million dog bites annually. The visible damage from a dog bite may be worse than that from a cat bite, but a cat bite often has consequences that are more serious. Whereas dogs' teeth tear skin, cats' teeth puncture it. Both dogs and cats have an unusual bacterium in their saliva that can infect the bite wound and cause more damage than the bite itself. Because of the tearing, a dog bite is more likely to bleed, thereby flushing out the harmful bacteria before they can cause an infection. With either injury, an emergency room visit for wound cleansing, antibiotic treatment, and tetanus prevention is wise.

By the way, bacteria in human saliva are far more infectious than those in dog and cat saliva and, if ignored, cause devastating infections. Most human bites result from fights, where a hapless tooth penetrates the skin of a landing fist. So use psychology and back away slowly from snarling humans as well.

Avoiding eye contact with snakes has not proven effective. The good news is that most snakes are not poisonous, and even poisonous snakes have bad days and do not inject venom with every strike. The treatment for snakebites has changed completely since you probably went to camp, so if you can no longer find or fit into your Scout uniform, your training needs updating. Intravenous administration of antivenin neutralizes the poison's toxicity and is usually the only treatment needed.

Other treatments are generally ineffective, if not dangerous. The old remedy of lancing the fang marks and sucking out the venom is only effective if done immediately after the bite, but even then the knife may permanently damage nearby tendons and nerves. So forget your snakebite kit unless you are venturing into the deep and hospital-sparse wilderness.

Pound for pound, the most devastating bite comes from a drab, yellow-tan little creature with a 1-inch leg span—the brown recluse spider. It has a dark brown, violin-shaped marking on its back and is found in the warmer regions of the United States. An enzyme that thwarts the body's effort to wall off the poison accompanies the toxin, so the damage spreads. Treatment is not entirely effective, and victims can lose patches of skin or even parts of digits. Fortunately, the spider is nocturnal and shy, so we rarely encounter one. It prefers dry, dark crannies like crawl spaces, garage corners, and dense shrubbery. So while cleaning neglected areas, it is smart to wear gloves, but shake them out first. Then at night, don't eat crispy treats in bed, since the crumbs may attract spiders. I'm not sure about ice cream.

Swine, seal, monkey, and camel bites have their unique features. Really! The average devotee of summer can usually avoid them, but don't forget the mosquito repellent.

JULY: LEARNED HAND, 1872-1961

Image a newborn burdened with the weight of three family surnames: Billings, Learned, and Hand. Add a hovering mother who wanted a fourth family name and a bookish, emotionally remote father who dies when the boy is 14. The young man studies philosophy at Harvard and then reluctantly chooses law, the family profession for generations. After that he lives with his mother until he is 30 and writes her thoughtful 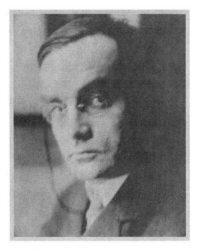 and nearly daily letters for the rest of her life.

This neurotic, insecure intellectual fails at lawyering but because of his recognized grasp of the law, is appointed to a judgeship at age 37. From this background, Hand rises to become, as *The New York Times* described, "the greatest jurist of his time," spending 25 years on the U.S. Court of Appeals. His balanced, probing, reasoned approach on the bench led to many influential decisions, especially those regarding personal freedoms. Law students today still study them thoroughly.

His last law clerk and recent biographer, Gerald Gunther, describes Hand as having "a deep rooted open mindedness and skepticism about his work, a capacity to doubt his own tentative conclusions and to insist on putting them to the test of the most rigorous analysis."

Hand's influence has exceeded that of many judges on the Supreme Court, a seat on which he quietly aspired to but for which he was passed over several times because of his political independence.

On a Sunday afternoon in 1944 in New York's Central Park, he gave a brief speech that vaulted him from a jurist respected within his profession to a nationally recognized intellectual. The occasion was the swearing-in ceremony for 150,000 naturalized citizens. Patriotism was rampant. America sensed the fortunes of war moving in the Allies' favor; D-Day, as it turned out, was two weeks off. Hand's 500-some words rival Lincoln's Gettysburg Address for their simplicity and eloquence. In conclusion he said:

> "What then is the spirit of liberty? I cannot define it; I can only tell you my own faith. The spirit of liberty is the spirit which is not too sure that it is right; the spirit of liberty is the spirit which seeks to understand the minds of other men and women; the spirit of liberty is the spirit which weighs their interests alongside its own without bias; the spirit of liberty remembers that not even a sparrow falls to earth unheeded; the spirit of liberty remembers that the spirit of Him, who, nearly two thousand years ago, taught mankind that lesson it has never learned, but has never quite forgotten: that there may be a kingdom where the least shall be heard and considered side by side with the greatest."

He then led the estimated million people assembled in the park and listening on speakers in the Pledge of Allegiance. This learned, self-doubting philosopher deserves a Fourth of July hand.

AUGUST: "TENNIS ELBOW? NO WAY. I DON'T PLAY."

Many of the muscles that control forearm and finger movements anchor to bone around the elbow. Most of the muscles that open the fingers and lift the wrist attach to the outside of the elbow, and those that close the fingers and flex the wrist attach to the inside. Activities requiring forceful repetitive gripping may irritate and slightly loosen the muscles from their bony anchor points and cause elbow pain. Tennis elbow is the common description for muscle irritation on the outside of the elbow. Golfer's elbow identifies the same condition on the inside of the elbow (near the funny bone).

You certainly do not have to play golf or tennis to get either condition. Carrying heavy shopping bags, laptop computer, or carry-on luggage, lifting a briefcase repeatedly over the console or into the backseat of a car, prolonged hammering, or nearly any other forceful, repetitive activity can cause symptoms, especially if you happen to be between 40 and 60.

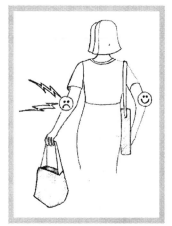

Once the muscle-bone junction becomes irritated, just light daily activities such as opening doors or brushing teeth may be enough to perpetuate the irritation. When the inflammation is severe, any finger or wrist motion may cause elbow agony.

Treatment includes anti-inflammatory medications and protecting the irritated area. The first means of protection is to stop aggravating the sore spot by using shoulder straps or wheeled luggage to transport laptops, shopping bags, carry-on luggage, and toolboxes. Sorry, but stopping the aggravators may also require a respite from golf, tennis, and weight lifting.

The second means of protection is regular use of a snugly applied Velcro hook and loop band around the forearm, just below the elbow. It serves as a shock absorber and dampens some of the irritating activity generated by wrist and finger motion. In recalcitrant cases, a wrist splint may help by even further slowing down activity in the offending muscles. Be prepared. It is going to take six to twelve months to feel better.

In the meantime, your friends and colleagues will tell you about a basketful of remedies—acupuncture, cortisone injection, blood injection, ultrasound, shock wave therapy, magnets, lasers—all expensive, none with proven effectiveness. The fountain of youth remains elusive, but rest and patience are usually rewarded with a gradual lessening of symptoms, at which time a stepwise return to a modest level of sport is appropriate. Consultation with a tennis or golf pro or personal trainer may help at this time.

Weekend warriors with symptoms persisting over a year usually benefit from surgery. Of course, the operation itself is a major irritation, and convalescence occurs over months, not days. Like other types of overuse problems, prevention or early treatment of tennis elbow is best. Do not ignore your body's plea to slow down when you are doing something that makes you hurt.

SEPTEMBER: THE FRUITS OF OUR LABORS

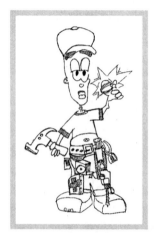

Labor Day officially honors working people. But rather than resting and reflecting, many people fill this extended, end-of-summer weekend with frenetic manual activity. Whether in the garage, garden, or garret, three straight days of home labor can take its toll on unconditioned, tender hands. Here are three reasons to wear work gloves.

Blisters, in essence, are burns. None of us would willingly burn our hands in a hot oven, but somehow we can get engrossed in chopping ivy, driving screws, or cutting miles of fabric and forget that the friction from tool handles can also burn. Only you can prevent blisters. Use gloves. Then you can probably keep working until your muscles ache!

If you do get a blister, at least stop the manual abuse before the blister opens. The superficial layer of blistered skin protects the deeper layers of skin from infection for at least a few days while the burn begins to heal. Whenever the blister does pop, carefully trim back the edges so that you can wash away dirt and bacteria. Then use a little antibiotic ointment, a Band-Aid adhesive strip, and a nice comfortable chair to plan your Thanksgiving weekend project.

So, you may ask, why don't full-time gardeners, mechanics, and carpenters get blisters even though they may go gloveless? Well, they do wear gloves of a sort—built-in gloves: calluses. Their hands, like everybody's feet, gradually become conditioned to friction by secreting a tough protective material called keratin. (Fingernails are also made of keratin.)

Calluses can provide leather-like protection, unless they get so thick that they crack, bleed, and get infected. Then, even regular tool users may wish they wore gloves more often.

Sanding down prominent calluses with a pumice stone prevents excessive buildup. This is easier when the calluses are soft after bathing or spending Labor Day in a Jacuzzi.

While blisters and calluses creep up slowly, thorns and splinters attack suddenly and without warning. Rose thorns, palm fronds, and cactus spikes all afford plants natural protection from weekend warriors and other predators. Splinters seem to come out of nowhere but are equally nasty. Again, gloves are the best defense. If the unpleasant thought of getting stuck is not sufficient motivation to wear gloves, consider this: Certain plants can deposit chemicals that keep your skin inflamed even after the spike is removed, and deep stabs with rose thorns may introduce fungal spores that set up housekeeping on your tendons—easy to prevent, difficult to treat. Don't take on Labor Day bare-handed.

OCTOBER: PUMPKIN CARVER'S FINGER

Each October, hand surgeons across the country are called to treat a serious and avoidable injury. We call it pumpkin carver's finger. Here are the ghoulish details.

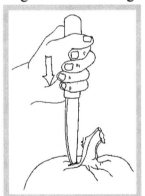

The enthusiastic vegetable-carving artist grasps the knife in a stabbing fashion. When the knife handle is slippery and the pumpkin offers unanticipated resistance, the carver's clenched hand slips forward onto the blade, slashing critical nerves and tendons where the fingers joint the palm. Despite even the best surgical repair and subsequent rehabilitation, full function rarely returns.

Are you safe if you just stop carving pumpkins? Not necessarily. This kind of knife injury happens all year, especially while someone is trying hastily to break apart pieces of frozen meat. Now that you know about the danger, don't stab frozen food—defrost it or call Domino's.

And back to pumpkin carving: Don't use kitchen knives. Various child-safe (and adult-proof) tools designed especially for pumpkin carving are commercially available. For the do-it-yourselfers, you can easily make one with a few

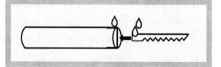

simple supplies from the hardware store. Start with a piece of broom handle or thick wooden dowel. Make it at least a foot long so the carver can control it with both hands. Saw a slit in one end and epoxy in a course-toothed saber saw blade.

Here's another safety tip for Halloween. Cut off the bottom of the pumpkin rather than the top. Then you can place your carved masterpiece over a lighted candle. This beats burning your hand by reaching down inside the pumpkin with a candle or match.

Happy tricking and treating. If somebody drops a bagel or an avocado in your goodie bag, read on. There is danger lurking.

PRACTICING SAFE BAGEL AND SAFE AVOCADO

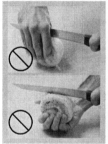 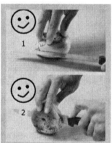

Bagel slicing often results in sliced fingers and palms. The knife teeters on the bagel's round and tough crust. The bagel wobbles on the cutting board. It slips. A trip to the emergency room annoyingly delays breakfast. To avoid risk to your skin, nerves, and tendons, lay the bagel down and press it firmly onto a flat surface with one hand. Hold the knife horizontally and saw at least halfway through. Then stand the bagel on edge, pinching the part already sliced, and complete the cut.

After cutting an avocado in half, that slippery pit resists extraction. So you stab it. The knifepoint slips off the pit and enters your palm. The most likely victim is a nerve to your fingers. Suddenly guacamole turns into a trip to the doctor with the probability of some permanent numbness on one or more fingertips despite the best microsurgical repair. Avoid this peril by hacking the pit lightly with the middle of the knife blade. Give the pit, now stuck to the knife, a slight sideways twist and flick it into the trash. *Olé!*

NOVEMBER: WEATHER ACHE

When Grandma's fingers begin to ache, she tells us rain is on the way. Is Grandma getting this information from her hands or has she been watching The Weather Channel on the sly?

Unstable atmospheric conditions are associated with areas of low air pressure. The extreme example is a hurricane. Meteorologists, sailors, and farmers among others keep track of barometric pressure for good reason. Even a less dramatic drop warns of coming rain or snow. Variations in atmospheric pressure make the mercury in a barometer go up or down. They also make our ears pop when we move vertically through the atmosphere on mountain roads and at the beginning and ending of plane flights. Identical, but more subtle changes in air pressure are at work in Grandma's joints.

Bone, obviously, is rigid, but tiny spaces, each containing a living cell, permeate it. These cells produce the calcium substance that accounts for the bone's strength. The water inside the bone cells is subject to atmospheric pressure just like everything else on earth. When the bone is not entirely normal, say in arthritic joints or for at least a year after a bone has been broken or operated on, these microscopic barometers act up and ache whenever the pressure changes.

In my hand surgery practice in southern California where it rains only in the winter, I have learned to expect some anxious phone calls after the first November storm moves in. I know I will hear from patients I have not seen in months. Perhaps they broke their wrist in May or had surgery in July, and then I discharged them several months later when they were feeling fine. Now they ache again and are worried that something is wrong. I explain it is just the sensitive barometers in their incompletely remodeled bone. For another year they can compete with Grandma for weather prediction.

DECEMBER: KITCHEN KNIGHTS

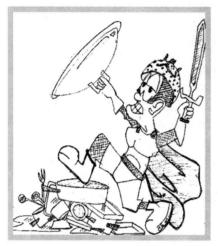

Boiling oil. Steel blades—some spinning. Rings of flaming gas. Most injuries are self-inflicted. Is this a Wagnerian opera? Medieval torture? No, it is just the kitchen. Regularly, our hands are at more risk here than anywhere else at home and especially so in December with family and friends pouring in for holiday feasts. How do you keep your hands safe?

The first risk is just getting ingredients into the kitchen. Nobody likes making extra trips in from the car with a week's worth of groceries. So we loop all those plastic bag handles over our fingers and struggle in. The weight from each bag compresses its flimsy handle strips into a narrow cord that digs in and exerts incredible pressure on the nerves at the bases of our fingers. Unless you want several numb fingers for a few months, haul in the bounty over several trips. Having avoided that problem, you are ready to cook. The injuries now come in two categories: burns and cuts. Again, avoidance is best.

Lifting a lid straight up from a boiling pan is a guaranteed way to steam your forearm. Protect yourself by tilting the top's handle toward you and using the lid as a shield as you remove it. Turn pan and skillet handles so they are not hanging off the front of the stove—that way they are safe from passersby snagging and dumping hot contents. Use both hands, well protected with pads or mitts, to lift any hot container. That way you have insurance against shifting contents, slipping grip, and unexpected weight or heat. A grease fire is especially scary. Snuff it out in place with baking soda or salt or by covering the pan with a cookie tray. Water does not choke off a grease fire's oxygen and only adds steam and splatter to the danger. It is worth holding a grease fire drill for young cooks.

Grease, steam, hot metal—whatever the delivery method—the results are identical: blisters and agony. Anything cold, ice or a pack of frozen veggies, for example, applied immediately and kept in place for 10 to 15 minutes not only counteracts the pain but also minimizes the tissue damage.

Strange at it may seem, sharp knives are less risky than dull ones. Here is the reason: The harder you have to push with a dull blade, the more likely the knife, the food, the cutting board, or all three are suddenly going to go somewhere unexpected. A wet slippery handle makes it even harder to control a dull knife. Even with a sharp knife firmly gripped in a dry hand, you do not want the cutting board or the food making a surprise move. Stabilize a wobbly cutting board by padding it on a dishtowel. Stabilize round or irregularly shaped fruits and vegetables by slicing off a section and facing the new flat surface on the board.

How do those TV chefs chop, dice, and slice at warp speed without adding their fingers to the recipe? They curl them under and hold the object to be cut with the very tips of their flexed fingers. Long nails here are a disadvantage. Their knuckles then serve as a fence to feel and control the blade's broad surface. The fingertips, closer to the board, are tucked safely away from the blade's advancing edge. It takes considerable practice, but mastery allows safe, speedy cutting while hardly looking.

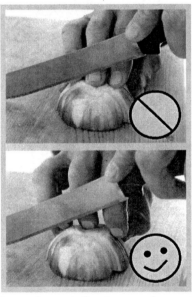

Bean dip, tuna fish, roasted almonds, pet food—maybe not holiday staples, but they all come in "convenience" cans with the little snap tabs and peel-back aluminum lids. Haste, wet hands, and inattention in any combination can suddenly cause that razor-sharp edge on the lid to slice a digital nerve. If that happens, you are likely to have some permanent numbness on your fingertip, even with the best microsurgical repair. Focus.

Another unsuspected culprit is the serrated metal edge on boxes of aluminum foil and plastic wrap. You are in a hurry, hands are wet, and the box slips and starts to fall. Do not grab at it—it is a flying saw blade.

Most cuts from broken kitchenware seem to occur during washing. Cups and glasses, maybe with microscopic cracks or tapped against the faucet, seemingly explode into gripping fingers. Scrub inside with a vegetable brush rather than manually forcing a sponge or cloth to the bottom. Also, rubber gloves provide an extra layer of protection. If your insecurity persists, the safest thing to make for a holiday dinner is reservations.

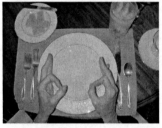

Here is one final tip for when you finally sit down at the banquet table. Sometimes the tableware is so crowded that it is hard to tell which bread plate and which drinking glass are yours. Fear no more. Use this simple digital mnemonic to set things straight. Put the tips of your index fingers on the tips of your thumbs. Note that your left hand makes a *b* and your right hand makes a *d*. The *b* is for bread (on your left) and the *d* is for your drink (on your right). Party on.

CHAPTER

7

Official

HANDS

I F YOU FASTENED A MAP ON THE WALL, STRETCHED A string between Memphis and Nashville, and then gave it a little slack, it would run right through Finger, Tennessee, population 279. On the application for a local post office, which was submitted in 1895, "Cash" was crossed out and "Finger" was inserted. Nobody presently knows why. The prevailing opinion among locals is that there was disagreement, heated discussion, and even finger-pointing during the naming process. Because there was a whole lot of finger shaking going on, somebody suggested memorializing the act. We can only surmise that they left in agreement, sealing the deal and parting with a handshake.

Hands have other official roles as well. "Raise your right hand and repeat after me" asks for a sign of sincerity, loyalty, and honesty at various swearing-in ceremonies. A salute signifies respect. Hands also figure into government-issued maps, coins, stamps, and even license plates. Let's explore.

SEALED WITH A SHAKE, OR A KISS

The custom of two people grasping right hands upon meeting, agreement, or farewell has ancient and uncertain origins. Quite likely, holding the weapon hand of one's enemy during a truce reduced the risk of a sudden change of heart. Similarly, extending an empty right hand would be a gesture of peaceful intentions 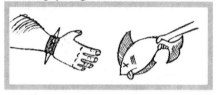 and good will. Regardless of intentions, however, Attila undoubtedly instantly killed anybody offering him a dead-fish handshake.

Today, handshakes come in many forms, with regional stereotypes. Midwesterners are accused of the longest, most vigorous shakes, reminiscent of pumping water on the farm. With a puritanical resistance to sensuality, easterners quickly squeeze and release. In Los Angeles, of course, style is everything—the delicately offered fingers; the two-handed shake with the left hand on hand, wrist, elbow, shoulder, or neck; the hand clasp as a prelude to cheek kissing.

Hand kissing has pretty well fallen out of vogue except in Dracula movies and among favor-seeking men who watch Dracula movies. The hand kiss is the equivalent of a handshake, except that deference to the kissee is implied. The kisser can imply great deference by kneeling rather than bowing but must be careful not to trip on his cape. Etiquette manuals differ as to whether the kisser should feign a kiss from several millimeters away, kiss his own thumb, or actually contact his dry lips lightly to the recipient's hand. Who knows where it has been? However, I digress.

Specialized handshakes may be as subtle as a members-only grasp of interlocking fingers or as flamboyant as a dance of rhythmic bumps, snaps, and slaps. The athletes' high-five most likely originated as a sign of agreement. Even 18th century literature refers to sealing a bargain by slapping hands.

How many hands do you shake in an eight-hour day at work? If it is over 14,000, you are good for the record book. New Mexico politician Bill Richardson currently holds the record at

13,392, which works out to one about every two seconds. Richardson crushed Teddy Roosevelt's 1907 record and ended his 2002 flesh-pressing quest by soaking his sore, stiff hand in a bucket of ice water.

Whether or not Richardson remembers the names of all he greeted, the handshake is a powerful social gesture. Having anything less than a normal hand to offer may lead a person to seek medical attention. Antiperspirant can help mildly sweaty palms. Hands that constantly drip moisture can be relieved with endoscopic surgery in the neck that divides the nerves that control sweating. Stiff fingers may send an unintended message. Sore joints or inflamed tendons may cause the recipient of a firm shake to wince or pull back, countering the intended message of friendship and accord. In many instances, hand therapy or surgery can reduce soreness and stiffness to restore a normal grip.

This age-old gesture of shaking hands, nevertheless, may be dying. With cell phone in one hand and a cup of latte in the other, modern warriors can only nod and hope to avoid being splashed. Coins and bank notes, however, will likely preserve the memory of this human gesture of accord far into the future. Friends of mine, all hand surgeons, have contributed the next three sections related to their personal passions for official hands. A display of my hand-related collecting passion will come later.

HANDS ON ANCIENT GREEK AND ROMAN COINAGE

Designs struck on metal discs of gold, silver, and bronze started in Lydia, what today is the western coast of Turkey. Coinage caused a revolutionary change in the way trade occurred, and its use spread rapidly throughout ancient Greece, which encompassed a wide region from present day France through Italy and Greece proper to the east in Turkey and Cyprus. In as little as 75 years, coins with designs specific to the city's issuing them were found throughout the Greek world. They standardized and streamlined trade. It is, after all, much easier to go to the market with a pocket full of silver coins than a few oxen. Coins were also a form of propaganda for their issuing city-states who used clever and artistic designs to promote themselves.

In some locations, huge numbers of coins were minted. Athens, arguably the most powerful of all ancient city-states, struck hundreds of thousands of coins all with the image of Athena, the goddess of wisdom, on one side and an owl on the other. This coin type was recognized throughout the ancient world and even imitated in certain parts. The number of coins struck by Alexander the Great during his conquest of the Mediterranean rivaled that of Athens.

As the political use of coinage developed, hundreds of large and small city-states of Greece began to strike their own coins with specific designs. The ability to issue one's own coinage imparted prestige and a sense of place during times of war and shifting alliances. The first designs on coins were crude, but as city-states chose to advance their cause, they began to hire better die engravers who had probably worked on jewelry, cameos, and metal art objects previously. A fascinating acceleration of the art of coin design took place based on the ensuing competition to produce the finest.

The designs found on the obverse (anvil side) and reverse (hammer side) of both ancient Greek and Roman coins are immensely varied. They encompass nearly every known animal, portraits of rulers, mythical Gods and creatures, and scenes from history. Hands also appeared on ancient coins, especially clasped hands, which symbolized unity and togetherness. In general, an individual hand on coins of the ancient Greeks was usually a symbol within a larger design.

One of the most famous Greek silver coins comes from the island of Aegina just off the coast of Athens and was struck circa 5th century B.C. It was one of the most widely circulated silver

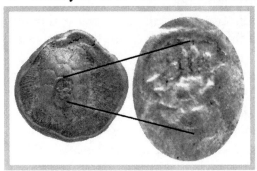

coins in all of ancient times and has been found in buried hoards from Africa to Turkey, indicating its wide use for trade. This particular example shows a land tortoise on the obverse with, at the high point of the shell, a countermark symbol of a hand. Traders used punches to countermark coins to check if they were solid silver rather than merely silver-coated bronze forgeries. Since the value of ancient coins related to the metal itself, it was important for traders to ensure the coins they were taking from far-off places were real. On this particular specimen, the trader marked the coin with a small human hand, confirming its value.

Another silver coin portrayed a large griffin with wings outstretched and a hand at its lower left. The coin was struck in the 5th century B.C. It is a tetradrachm, one of the largest denominations of ancient times. The hand in this design may have been the local magistrate's mark or even that of the die engraver.

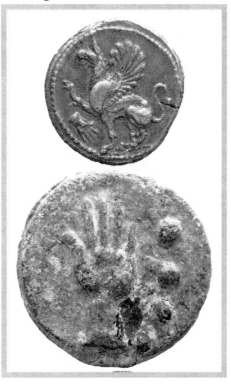

Around the 3rd century B.C., Rome was beginning to form its own power base. A common coinage of their early years was termed Aes Grave. These were very large cast bronze coins featuring different, somewhat crude designs. A spectacular example of this type of coinage depicted a large, well-formed hand with outstretched finger and three small dots alongside. The reverse side of this coin also carries the identical hand design.

Over the ensuing several centuries, power shifted entirely to Rome. Emperors, including Julius Caesar, Nero, and Hadrian, ruled the empire, which during its height stretched from Great Britain across Europe to Africa and the East, much as the lands of Alexander the Great did 500 years before.

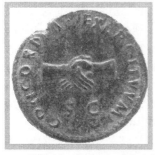 Coins during the time of Emperor Nerva commonly included clasped hands as a central motif. This large bronze coin, struck around 97 A.D., features two clasped hands on its reverse, signaling unity, which Nerva did not particularly enjoy during his reign.

Hands as an outreach of the human soul impacted the ancients as they do today. For the world's far-slung traders and merchants, the designs on these trusted tokens were symbolic of the issuing government's good will. (copyright *Arnold-Peter C. Weiss, MD*)

HANDS ON BANK NOTES

When toting bags of heavy coins became burdensome and risky, governments developed bank notes, which represented the coins or the silver and gold from which the coins were made. After users became comfortable with that leap of faith, governments quit backing bank notes with precious metals and based the currency only on the reputation and the strength of the country's economy. As with coins, bank notes have become miniature works of art as well as legal tender. Although they often depict the country's leader, hands have found their way onto paper money just as they did onto coins, but now with finer detail, shading, and even color.

Hands joined in friendship and unity are again common themes. For instance, this El Salvador 50-peso note from 1897 features two hands shaking. In 1967 Singapore released a 10-dollar note that shows the clasping of four hands, each a different color and representing the nation's ethnic groups--Chinese, Malay, Indian, and all others.

Portugal has a 5,000-escudo note, released in 1987, that has six hands linked by chains and ropes that represent the fraternal binding of its six historical provinces.

Not seen on coins because of the detail required, hands depicted on bank notes commonly provide sustenance or protection. The 1994 Mexican 10-peso note has a pair of hands

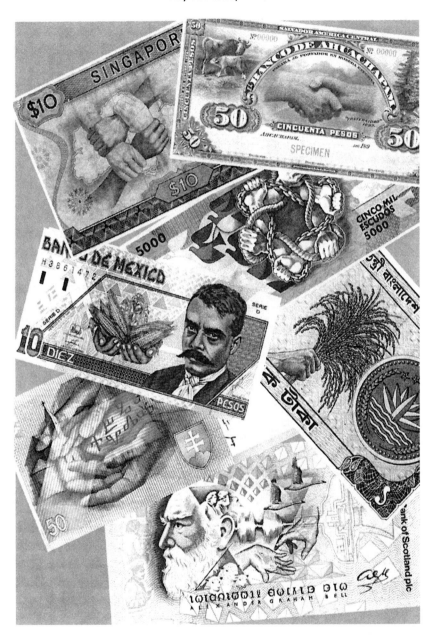

holding corn, essential to the national diet. Similarly, the 1973 Bangladesh one-taka note shows a hand holding rice, another regional staple. Slovakia's 10-korun note from 1993 features two hands with the first seven letters of the Old Slavic alphabet between them, representing the gift that two saints brought to the ancient Slavs. The medieval church also shown on the note recalls the dawn of Christianity in Slovakia.

Busier yet, this 1997 one-pound note from Scotland marks the 150th anniversary of the birth of Alexander Graham Bell. Two hands represent sign language and the phonetic alphabet as a reminder that Bell was a teacher of the deaf as well as an inventor. (*Bill Myers, MD*)

HANDS OFFICIALLY STAMPING OUT DISEASE

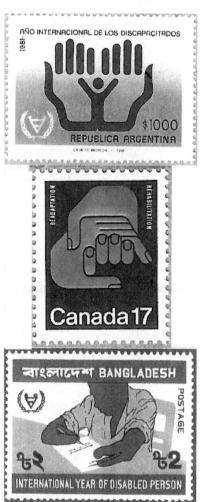

Although postage stamps are generally smaller than bank notes in physical size and face value, they are the hands-down winners for expressing multitudes of sentiments on governmental art. Appearing on thousands of stamps worldwide, hands are common motifs, often conveying abstract and noble messages of cooperation or protection. They also hold torches and flags, vote, reach up, and break chains. Other postal images simply celebrate the versatility of hands for work and recreation as well as commemorate various individuals, events, and organizations. Examples of these miniature masterpieces appear throughout the book because they beautifully illustrate various topics. Here are stamps and hands that relate to medicine and health. They come from the collection of Dr. Terry Light.

120

Many countries published stamps in 1981 to recognize the International Year of the Disabled. Here are three of the most graphic. The first, from Argentina, is highly stylized, shows a pair of hands nurturing an individual with hands raised in a presumed gesture of success or victory. The second one, from Canada and somewhat stylized, depicts a universally understood graphic of caring. You may find the third, from Bangladesh, grotesque and shocking in its realism. Perhaps from an industrial or farm accident or from war, this man is missing both hands and has had operations to create some pinch function between the bones in his forearm. This permits some grasp and pinch function without the need for prostheses, which may be in short supply in underdeveloped countries. Although perhaps shocking, this image certainly underscores the often-neglected needs of the disabled.

These two stamps depict diseased hands. The first is from Austria and shows the joint swelling and pain in the hand related to rheumatoid arthritis. The cane illustrates the demand that these patients put on their hands for weight bearing and balance during ambulation. The other stamp, from the Malagasy Republic (presently Madagascar), shows hands destroyed by leprosy. The offending bacteria destroy nerves, leaving the fingers without sensation and vulnerable to unfelt trauma and infections, which eventually lead to their destruction. Unpleasant thoughts to be sure, but for the mere cost of a postage stamp, the plight of these people can be publicized worldwide.

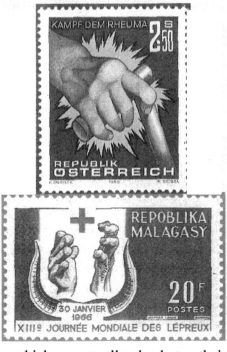

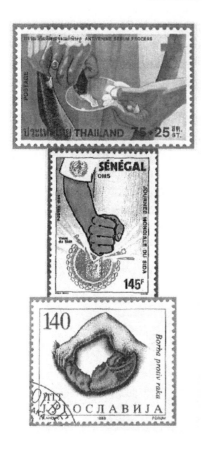

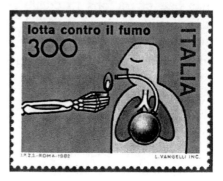

The third theme relates to treatments for various conditions: Thailand, poisonous snakebites; Senegal, AIDS; and Yugoslavia, cancer.

The final motif is a hand actually *contributing* to disease. In doing so, however, the overall health message is dramatic.

MARKING THE GOODS

Long before the existence of coins, bank notes, and stamps, ancient potters and stonemasons made distinctive marks on their handcrafted goods so others could identify each object's source. Today, businesses seek memorable marks that promote a positive image. Features of a good trademark include its ability to remain recognizable in black and white and in varying degrees of enlargement or reduction. Hence the graphics must be bolder and simpler than postage stamps or bank notes. Trademarks involving hands frequently appear on the stationery of hand surgeons and hand therapists as well as hospitals. The message is typically caring.

Outside the health professions, hands also appear in logos, and they convey one of four basic messages.

The first is the hand at work. The message is simple and concrete and testifies to the hand's versatility, dexterity, and strength.

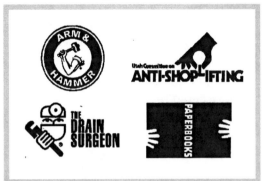

In the second and third messages, the symbol expands an actual manual activity to represent an endeavor of body and mind: the hand providing protection and the hand offering friendship and cooperation.

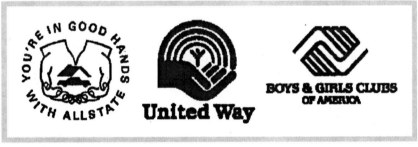

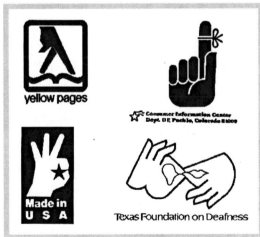

The fourth message is the hand as an abstract sign. This is the most interesting and complex, since here the hand's position, unrelated to any concrete manual activity, conveys the message. These are among the many gestures of which the hand is capable.

An official gesture, to be explored next, is the military salute.

CLEAN LACE AND DIRTY PALMS

It is time for a quiz. How did saluting get started?

A. Roman soldiers shaded their eyes from intense light beaming from their superiors' eyes.

B. While passing one another on horseback, armored knights raised their visors with their right hands to allow for mutual recognition.

C. One day at a tournament, a contestant shielded his eyes from the dazzling beauty of some fair maiden watching from the stands.

D. Removing one's head gear repeatedly in the presence of an officer became impractical, so a hand movement became the acceptable substitute.

E. At a time when assassins used knives, one could only approach a public official with the right hand raised and obviously empty.

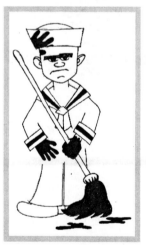

The origin of the salute is lost in time, and although all of the above theories have their proponents, some documentation actually supports D. Out of concern for disfiguring the hat or dirtying its lace with repeated acknowledgement of an officer's presence, the Royal Scots issued new orders in 1762. A soldier needs only to briskly raise the back of his hand to his hat when passing an officer. This gesture became the standard "open hand" salute of British troops where the palm faces forward and is visible to the recipient.

Because palms were often stained from the tar and pitch used to seal their wooden sailing ships, the British Navy adopted a slightly different salute. By rotating the hand 90 degrees so that the palm faced down, the salutee was spared the insult of viewing grime. This floated across the Atlantic and became the standard American salute.

The civilian equivalent to the military salute is the hand-over-heart posture used during solemn patriotic moments. Regardless of their murky origins, all of these hand gestures signify respect, and somewhere along the line, military uniform designers showed respect for the troops by dropping the lace.

GENERAL HAND

One of the first to live the American dream, Edward Hand started life abjectly impoverished in Ireland and ended as a Pennsylvania gentleman farmer and confidant of George Washington. Hand attended Trinity College in Dublin and studied medicine, which at that time consisted of only several courses in the college curriculum. To practice medicine thereafter, a 5-year apprenticeship was standard, and Hand chose to do it as a surgeon's mate in the British army. He was shipped to the American frontier (near present-day Pittsburgh) where the presence of a military force was intended to protect settlers from Indian attacks.

Hand completed his service in 1774. He settled in Lancaster, Pennsylvania, to practice medicine amid growing colonial unrest. Within months following Paul Revere's famous ride, Hand accepted a commission in the Continental Army. In the hills around Boston, the riflemen under his command strengthened earthen defenses (breastworks) while evading British cannon fire. "I kept men to look out and we constantly fell in our ditch at the flash [of the cannon fire]. Lads indeed not accustomed to such music were at first a little shy of working on the breast works, which obliged me to show them the example and work very hard which soon learned them to evade and despise the cannon."

Hand's leadership abilities and his knowledge of British military ways caught the eye of General George Washington, and Hand was rapidly promoted. Hand gave outstanding service against the British at battles of Long Island, White Plains, Trenton (where he crossed the Delaware with Washington), and Princeton. His right eye was wounded in an early battle, and portraits of Hand show only his left profile.

Upon promotion to brigadier general, Hand was ordered to western Pennsylvania where he had originally been garrisoned in the British army. Now, his assignment was to protect the colonialists against the British and Indians as well as settlers who remained loyal to the Crown. Results here were mixed as they were during a subsequent campaign to destroy Indian villages, livestock, and crops in central New York. The logic was that Indians needing to restore their food supply would be less likely to side with the British and fight the colonialists.

Alexander Hamilton felt slighted when Washington picked Hand in 1780 to become adjutant general of the Continental army. In this role as chief administrative officer, Hand again distinguished himself. He supervised a reorganization of the army despite the unwillingness of Congress and the states to adequately supply the troops. Hand and his staff later prepared the "Regulations for the Service of the Siege" that led to Cornwallis's surrender at Yorktown.

Hand returned to Lancaster to be with his family and practice surgery, but his eyesight was poor. He was selected to represent Pennsylvania in the United States Congress where he contributed to congressional decisions on matters of Western lands, now having a 20-year off-and-on exposure to the region. He later campaigned for Lancaster to become the first capital of the United States, but New York City won out. Hand and Washington remained friends and visited back and forth at Mount Vernon and at Hand's home in Lancaster, Rock Ford.

Hand died at age 58 of cholera—a long dream away from his native Ireland but of a disease well known to his childhood.

BIRD-IN-HAND, PENNSYLVANIA

Two Pennsylvania road surveyors debated whether to spend the night at a local inn or ride seven miles west to Lancaster. One observed, "A bird in the hand is worth two in the bush," and so they stayed put. From that decision, their chosen inn and then the whole village became known as Bird-in-Hand. Edward Hand would have traveled the pike from Lancaster to Philadelphia beginning about 40 years after the road was surveyed and built.

He would have passed through Bird-in-Hand and near or through other colorfully named villages such as Blue Ball, White Horse, Fertility, Intercourse, and Paradise. Today the route is a designated scenic byway and the population of Bird-in-Hand is several hundred.

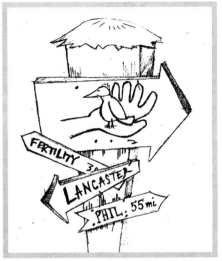

If you wanted to take a cross-country official hand tour, start in Bird-in-Hand, Pennsylvania, and head south to Palm Beach. On the way back, turn left at Left Hand, West Virginia, and then point toward Finger, Tennessee. Next stop would be Hand County, South Dakota, named for George H. Hand. Today, there are fewer than three people per square mile living in Hand County, so let *me* tell you about George before we continue on to California.

HAND COUNTRY

George H. Hand was born in 1837 in Akron, Ohio. He studied law with his father, practiced briefly in Wisconsin, Missouri, and Iowa, and then served in the Union forces for a year at the end of the Civil War. In 1865, Hand moved to Dakota Territory, where several months later he was appointed U.S. district attorney. After

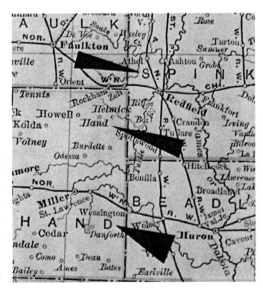

four years he resigned to practice law with S.L. Spink, who was territorial secretary.

During this time, the legislature divided the territory into counties and named two adjacent ones Hand and Spink. George Hand later served ably as territorial secretary and then as acting governor just before South Dakota attained statehood in 1889. Postal records indicate that until 1905 there was also a town named Hand located in Hand County, as seen on this 1895 map.

LICENSE TO SPEAK

Our cross-country official hand tour ends in Palm Springs, California. Palm Desert and Twenty Nine Palms are nearby, nearly close enough to walk to, but Californians are car crazy, so we drive everywhere and watch for vanity license plates. The California Department of Motor Vehicles promotes this amazing form of public art--personalized license plates--and challenges creativity by limiting the expression to seven letters. Have you spotted any of these?

Some license plates describe the car.
RTHNDDR HNDBLT HNDEDWN SORTHMB
HNDSOFF ELBOWRM

Others say something about the driver.
OWTAHND AHNDFUL HNDCFME

These might be seen at the gym or playing field.
HNDBALL HNDSPRG LFTHNDR GR8HNDS

The doctors' parking lot is good hunting.
HANDDOC HANDFXR HANDMD N2HNDS N2ELBOS
IFXHNDS STDYHND GDHNDS SZRHNDS

How about outside the hardware store or lumberyard?
SOHANDY MYTHNDY HANDYMN HANDYWMN
HNDYMAM HNDYLDY

Sweethearts also have their say.
HNDNHND HNDNHRT

Imagine a garage with these cars side by side.

IDLHNDS	BZFNGRS
FNGRNLS	GRNTHMB
LNDAHND	HLPNHND
HVEHNDS	LTFNGRS
HANDSON	HNDSOFF
IRONHND	GLDFNGR
NOHANDS	BOTHAND

How about three cars abreast on the freeway?

HND2MTH	PANHNDL	MTHAND
COOLHND	WRMHNDS	HOTHNDS
BIGHAND	BAREHND	BADHAND
FARMHND	RANCHND	COWHAND
LTFNGRS	HNDZUP	RDHNDD

Finally, match these plates with their owners' occupations.

HNDTLKR	bookie
1STHAND	personal assistant
THMBSUP	reporter
HNDCAPR	sign language interpreter
HNDMDN	movie critic

GVURSLFAHND--then ON2BEUTFLHNDS, where I will explain a major contribution to hand elegance from the automotive industry.

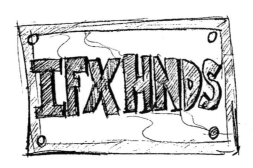

CHAPTER

8

Beautiful

HANDS

WILLIAM STEWART HALSTED WAS 37 YEARS OLD AND a dynamo of energy and ideas when he became Surgeon-in-Chief at Johns Hopkins Hospital in Baltimore upon its opening in 1889. At that time, general anesthesia was less than 50 years old and bacteria had only more recently been recognized as a cause of disease.

Over the next 30 years, Dr. Halsted and his protégés made monumental improvements in surgical concepts and techniques and brought surgery into the modern era. He thereby earned the epitaph, "Father of American Surgery."

How then could the development of surgical gloves stem from warm concerns of love rather than cool surgical reasoning? In that era, doctors recognized the benefits of scrubbing their skin before surgery, but they operated with bare hands. The surgical instruments were boiled or baked and then immersed in carbolic acid to ensure sterility. It was the surgical nurse's responsibility to pick instruments out of the carbolic acid jars and trays and hand them to the surgeon.

Dr. Halsted was distressed to see a severe rash on the head surgical nurse's hands and forearms produced by this practice. He asked the Goodyear Rubber Company to make two pairs of thin rubber gloves for her. These worked so well that other members of the surgical team began wearing them for protection from the harsh sterilizing solution. It was truly an afterthought that gloving also would reduce risk of infection. Over the following ten years, caps, masks, sterile gowns with long sleeves, and sterile gloves slowly became universally accepted operating room apparel.

Whether Caroline Hampton was charmed by Dr. Halsted's concern for her rash or whether the surgeon was attracted by his nurse's hands, now restored to their former beauty, is uncertain. At any rate, they married. What else can we learn about splendiferous hands?

FINGERNAILS: BLESSINGS OR CURSES?

Manicurists say they are blessings-- nails are their livelihood. Repair people who have just smashed their thumbs with hammers say curses. Overall, when well formed, clean and maybe painted nails are crown jewels. When disfigured or painful, they disturb physical and mental well-being far out of proportion to their size.

Fingernails are also tiny historical archives. Depending on the length of your nails, the edge you file or clip today reflects your health and diet from four to eight months ago. If somebody was trying to poison you back then or you were taking medications, your nails know. Also, a severe illness slows nail production; when health and nail production are restored, a transverse groove appears similar to a tree's seasonal growth ring.

Lizards and cats use their nails to climb trees—claws. Horses walk on theirs—hooves. Our nails stabilize the skin on the extreme tips of our fingers for manipulating tiny objects with precision, for instance picking up and threading a needle. They are also useful for scratching, scraping, and guitar playing.

The factory that produces this miraculous little tool starts almost a quarter of an inch back from the cuticle. Specialized skin cells there in the nail fold secrete a protein called keratin, which hardens. Today's secretion pushes yesterday's production out the door causing slow longitudinal growth—about an eighth of an inch a month. Perhaps a fourth to a half of this growth is worn away with daily use. A whole industry is ready to help us remove the remainder. It is possible to cut the nail so short that the corners plough into the skin as the nail plate relentlessly pushes forward. Ingrown fingernails are not nearly as common as ingrown toenails but certainly get the owner's attention when they occur.

Various lumps and bumps can form around and under the nail just like anywhere else on the skin. Two come immediately to mind. One is common and the other is life-threatening. First the common one.

With wear and tear in the joint closest to the nail, bone spurs can form. Such a spur can irritate the surrounding soft tissue, which causes a cyst to form. The cyst can raise and thin the skin, break open and drain, and even press on the nail production area to cause a longitudinal trough in the nail. Effective treatment for this constellation of findings is a minor surgical procedure to remove 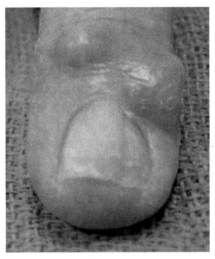 the bone spur. Once the irritating source is gone, the other problems resolve.

Cancers can form anywhere, but sometimes their growth around the nail is overlooked. This may happen because we become tolerant of the nail's slow growth and of the tendency to have repeated minor fingertip injuries. Areas that are repeatedly 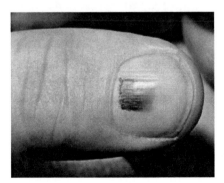 treated as warts and do not heal deserve a biopsy as does any other nonhealing area. The same holds true for discolored areas underneath the nail that cannot be clearly attributed to a recent injury or that do not move outward with the advancing nail plate over several months.

What else can go wrong with fingernails? Lots. There are whole books devoted to nail disorders—most are systemic conditions. The nails are a reflection of the skin, and the skin is a reflection of the whole body. Chronic skin conditions as well as essential nutrient deficiencies, hormonal imbalances, and certain heart and lung disorders can cause nail changes. Fungus can creep under the nail plate causing detachment and discoloration. Fungus can also invade the nail fold through a break in the cuticle and slowly irritate the surrounding skin. Your family doctor or dermatologist is best suited to manage these chronic conditions. That is, all chronic conditions except nail length over 12 inches, where perhaps a psychiatrist should get involved.

Emergency rooms and hand surgeons are the best resources for treating acute changes around the nail. These include car door slams, splinters, hammer strikes, and sudden signs of infection. Early treatment for nail-bed lacerations and fingertip injuries offers the best chance of maximal restoration of function and appearance—admirable qualities of these crown jewels.

STAINING AND PAINTING

A tall shrub known scientifically as *Lawsonia inermis* grows in subtropical bands both above and below the equator from the Mediterranean east to the Pacific Rim. Ancient men in those regions may have been annoyed that the crushed leaves from this plant stained their palms orange, but the women saw it differently—the potential for decorative art. When these leaves are dried, ground, and mixed with a little lemon juice, the paste can be applied artfully to the skin to stain decorative patterns. It is known as *henna* in the Middle East and *mehndi* in India and by a variety of other names in other areas. The different names imply that many cultures discovered henna's glories independently.

Throughout the regions where the plant grows and transcending those area's cultures and religions, henna is associated with celebrations—especially weddings. Henna decorations may have started at a time when other forms of bridal adornment were scarce. Henna is applied for luck and joy as well as beauty. The bride typically receives the most extensive and elaborate adornment, which in some cultures may take five days to apply. Grooms and even wedding guests often join the festivities. Henna has become associated with any joyful occasion—religious days, new years, battle victories, births, birthdays, and circumcisions (well, at least for bystanders). Henna and champagne seem to have the same connotation as "party time."

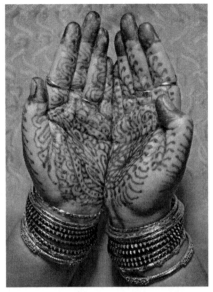

The most enduring henna decorations are on the palms and soles where the henna binds particularly well to the thicker skin. Depending on the quality of the paste and the length of time it is left in place, the reddish-brown color can last from several weeks to several months. The skin is always renewing itself, so gradually the staining fades away as the older stained cells come to the surface and flake away. Then it's time for another celebration!

Although body decoration with henna has strong regional origins, the equally ancient art of fingernail painting was practiced in locations as geographically diverse as China, Egypt, and Peru. In Egypt, men and women alike had painted nails, and the darker the color, the higher the social status. Ingredients naturally varied by region but included egg white, gelatin, beeswax, and ground-up orchid, rose, and impatiens petals for color. Polished and tinted nails held sway for centuries before painted nails again became trendy in the 1920s, first in France, then in America, where there was a happy confluence between the flashy fashions and the development of automotive enamels in colors other than black. Artificial nails and acrylic nails followed. Fine brushes, glitter, appliqués, and special techniques offer further embellishments for these tiny canvases.

RINGS AND RING INJURIES

Rings symbolize friendship, love, engagement, and marriage. Let's explore their history, appeal, and dangers. Earliest rings come from the tombs of ancient Egypt. Hieroglyphs on massive pure gold rings denoted their owner's name and titles. These rings distinguished royalty from other classes, who wore rings of silver, bronze, glass, pottery, ivory, amber, or stone.

This distinction of authority and class extended to Roman times, when slaves were forbidden to wear rings, citizens wore rings of iron, and public officials wore gold. Lower-ranking officials, however, were permitted this privilege only while performing public duty.

Giving a ring to mark a betrothal stems from Roman times. Initially plain iron rings charmed the ladies, but gold became customary during the 2nd century. Gold marriage rings stem from the 5th century.

Jewelers were apparently slow to recognize the potential, since it was another 700 years before the custom of decorating engagement rings with gems developed.

Rings are powerful forces in folklore and mythology, especially so in Wagner's four-opera series, *The Ring of the Nibelung*. With themes taken from Norse and Teutonic mythology, this epic saga recounts the downfall of all who possessed "the ring," which gave its owner unlimited wealth and power over gods and men.

Besides conveying messages of power and social and marital status, rings through the ages have identified popes, archbishops, Freemasons, fraternity brothers, high school classmates, the wearer's birth month, and championship team members.

In addition to being symbolic, rings can also be functional. Beginning in the 15th century, signet rings engraved with a badge or trademark were used to authenticate letters and documents when pressed into soft sealing wax. A small key fixed to the ring with a pivot avoided that timeless problem of misplacement.

Poison rings had some popularity in Roman times. Pliny recorded that a wearer, to escape torture, "broke the gem of his ring in his mouth and died immediately."

The medieval *ring of death* held a reservoir of poison, a concealed spring, and a hollow point capable of imparting a fatal scratch during a seemingly friendly handshake.

Modern rings also present some hazards, not deadly, but nonetheless unexpected and troubling. When injury to the wrist, hand, or finger causes swelling, a ring can constrict circulation. Immediately after any such injury, all rings, bracelets, and watches should be removed until the swelling subsides.

In addition, gold and silver are excellent conductors of electricity, so anyone working around unshielded electric components wisely removes rings to avoid becoming part of the circuit. Rings are especially risky during a jump or fall if the ring catches on a high, sharp edge and holds the finger behind. Rings should definitely be removed, for instance, before slam dunking or climbing over chain-link fences. Those frequently exposed to such hazards (such as construction workers) and those to whom such an injury would be career ending (such as musicians) should consider having their rings notched and weakened or not wear rings at all. Then if snagged, the ring will break at one of the concealed notches rather than jerking the finger.

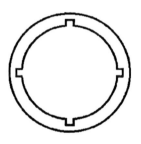

Less traumatic but still important are the emotional pains of getting rings over enlarged knuckles. Almost any ring can be removed without cutting it by using the soapy string technique.

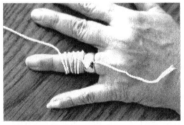

Take two to three feet of cotton string, tease one end under the ring and wrap the remaining string snugly around the finger. Then unwind the string, holding onto the end previously placed under the ring. The string gently guides the skin under the ring without bunching it up and slowly walks the ring over the enlarged knuckle.

Then of course, rings large enough to fit over the knuckle may be too loose at the finger's base. Teenage girls traditionally use tape to make the ring smaller. Jewelers can offer permanent

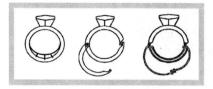

solutions, sometimes by just stretching the band, sometimes by using unseen mechanical contrivances.

HAND MODELING

Do you receive frequent, unsolicited compliments on the appearance of your hands? Could you completely shun sports, gardening, and household chores? If so, then you may wish to investigate the field of body parts modeling.

Believe it or not, those hands pouring Pepsi on television and the fingers in magazines and catalogues caressing soap, styling jewelry, and even gripping hammers are not just anybody's. They all belong to hand models. Such models get paid hundreds of dollars per hour to have their hands photographed for promotional and educational presentations and even for feature films. The leading man may have the perfect face and physique, but his hands may not make the grade for close-up shots. The body parts model lends perfect stand-in hands, and viewers never know.

You don't have glamorous hands? Don't despair. Hands suitable for a Chanel perfume ad would look ridiculous demonstrating table saws. There are calls for athletic, executive, blue collar, ethnic, and mature hands, both male and female, to name a few character types.

The hands that get the good parts are generally well proportioned with straight, symmetrical fingers. Smooth skin and a relative lack of hair, especially for female hands, are pluses. Perfect cuticles are important as are the absence of paper cuts, garden scratches, and similar daily insults.

Top hand models protect their hands fervidly, wearing gloves day and night, year round. A finger bullied by basketballs, cat claws, or household cleanser disables a hand model as quickly as laryngitis sidelines a singer.

The successful model's hands not only have to look right, they have to act right. They have to tell a story, hold a product in a natural and expressive manner, and demonstrate character (sometimes repeatedly for hours) while camera angles, lighting, and background are adjusted. During breaks, hand models check any make-up used to mask minor blemishes, stretch to relax tense muscles, and elevate their hands to flatten veins.

If you don't think you can persuade your spouse to shoulder all household chores so you can pursue your hand-modeling career, there may still be hope for you in pictures. The field of specialty-part modeling also has need for perfect teeth, sexy lips, beautiful eyes, great legs, and stylish feet.

COSMETIC HAND SURGERY

Once their other body parts have drunk deeply from the fountain of youth (cosmetic surgeon's office), the hands of age-conscious individuals can still reveal an unhappy truth: advancing years. The telltale signs include thin skin with dark blotches draped loosely over the metacarpals, prominent veins, and enlarged finger joints. Office procedures to conceal the evidence include sclerotherapy, chemical peels, bleaching creams, microdermabrasion, and laser skin resurfacing. Surgical procedures include vein stripping and fat cell injections. Before you dip your hands in the fountain of youth, however, here are several thoughts.

First, know that I am an orthopedic surgeon. We tend to focus on making things work. Plastic surgeons are well trained to consider aesthetics. Hand surgery needs both and involves both, but when it comes down to having my cake or eating it, I always vote for function first and then maximizing appearance. We normally take function for granted, especially while staring wistfully at our aging hands. But if the skin was rendered wrinkle free at the expense of being able to stretch sufficiently to make a tight fist, we would be unhappy. Also, anybody can easily dwell on their hands' imperfections both in public and in private, whereas it takes a mirror to examine one's face or body contours with equal scrutiny. Next, youth has not always been venerated as it currently is in American culture. The tide may well turn as the Baby Boomers move into their 60s and 70s. It may become cool to keep time with the Beatles by snapping arthritic fingers.

Gloves may again become fashionable, possibly just because they have been out of vogue for decades, and possibly because some trend-setting Boomer defines a new, "concealed" look.

Still not convinced? The treatments are expensive, sometimes costing thousands of dollars, and insurance does not cover them. Even if the skin looks better, thickened joints in otherwise serviceable fingers are still tell-tale signs for which there is no medical or surgical remedy. For skin blemishes, opaque creams can tone down discolorations effectively and economically. Rings can be modified to fit over thickened joints and may selectively attract the viewer's eye. The same goes for well-groomed nails. A cheery outlook, interest in new ideas and activities, and good posture also convey an image of health and vigor. Sunblock at any age is a wise idea.

I regularly look at hands that span nearly a 100-year age range. Overall, I like hands that reflect the integrity and character of their owner. They have stories to tell, maybe long stories. These hands of character don't reveal age, rather experience and wisdom. No cosmetic hand surgery for me. That's my two bits worth. Oops, I just revealed my age, even with my hands out of sight.

As beautiful as the hand is at all ages and in repose, it is at its best when in motion, and for that we thank its inner workings. Two examples follow.

THE SECRET JOINT

No, the secret joint is not Hernando's Hideaway, it is in your forearm. To get to the secret joint, put your elbows tightly against your sides and hold your hands in front of you. Turn one palm up to check for rain. Turn the other palm down ready for the keyboard. Now reverse your hands' positions.

What happened? Your elbows didn't open or close. Your wrists didn't bend frontward or backward. Yet the position of your hands changed dramatically. Palm-up activities include baby cradling and face washing. Palms need to turn down for writing, playing piano, pushing through doors, and waving. Your hand needs to turn smoothly from a palm down position when the spoon is in the soup to a palm up position by the time the spoon reaches your mouth. Otherwise you make a mess. Also, driving a screw is nearly impos-sible without forearm rotation.

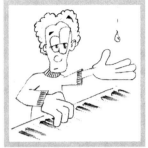

To understand the secret joint, cross your fingers. That is similar to your two forearm bones in the palm-down position. Now uncross them. That is similar to the forearm bones in the palm-up position. Forearm rotation is slightly more complicated, however, because as one forearm bone crosses over the other, it also rotates. If your fingers could do that, one fingernail would be facing up and the other facing down when you had them crossed.

So the two forearm bones (radius and ulna for the anatomy nuts) have contact surfaces with each other near the elbow and again near the wrist. Both portions of this forearm joint and everything in between have to work together to achieve rotation. By the way, there are also two bones in our leg reaching from knee to ankle, but these two are naturally stuck to each other pretty well, which means we cannot rotate our leg to point our toes backwards.

What happens if the forearm bones get stuck? The opportunities for them to do this are considerable. Any dislocation or sprain of the elbow or wrist or any break in either the radius or ulna puts forearm rotation at risk; and occasionally, a child is born with the two forearm bones fused together. To an extent, you can compensate for lack of palm-down motion by raising your elbow. To see what I mean, put your elbow against your side with your thumb pointing up. Now lift your elbow away from your side and note that your palm faces down. There is no contortion short of lying on your side, however, that will get the palm to face up when the secret joint is stiff. People find the inability to rotate their forearm extremely annoying, not only when trying to eat, but also when receiving change. Patients who cannot turn their palms up tell me that they ask the grocery clerk to put the change in the bag, and they ask the man at the toll booth to throw the coins in the backseat.

Hand surgeons and hand therapists take great pains to keep the forearm from getting stiff after an elbow or wrist injury. We also have some modestly effective means of surgically restoring rotation after injury to the forearm bones.

I guess I should not be surprised by people's response when I tell them that I am a hand surgeon. Since many people have never encountered a problem with their hands, I often see confused looks sweep across their faces when I tell them what I do. Their expression says they are asking themselves, "What could possibly go wrong that could keep a doctor busy doing just hands?" Maybe I should raise my eyebrows mysteriously and whisper, "The secret joint, for one thing."

When somebody is born with the two forearm bones fused together and preventing rotation, nobody may notice for years. Sometimes a high school coach or a piano teacher is the first to notice that the person moves the hand awkwardly. Up to that point, the family never realized that the secret joint was missing. The lesson here is that each of us uses whatever is available, but if we are missing something without knowing it, we find a way to get along. This message works for the secret joint and maybe for life in general.

BEAUTY IN NO MAN'S LAND

Today, the politically correct expression would be "no person's land" but such issues were not on Dr. Sterling Bunnell's mind in the early half of the 20th century when he applied this term to tendon injuries in the hand. Understanding no man's land and the considerable ingenuity and effort to surmount the difficulties encountered there go a long way toward clarifying the beauty of the normally functioning hand, its seemingly effortless grace and versatility, and the difficulties of managing tendon injuries in this area.

The motor units that allow us to make a fist start as muscles near the elbow and gradually transition into tendons, about the diameters of wooden pencils, which pass sequentially through the wrist, palm, and fingers. Similar to the way ferrules on a fishing pole control a fishing line's movement in any direction except back and forth along the pole, there are a series of arch-like bands beginning in the palm and continuing nearly to the fingertips. Each band is attached to an underlying bone and makes a tunnel through which the tendons pass. When the muscle in the forearm contracts, the tendon glides through this series of tunnels and draws the finger into a fist, just like an angler reeling in a fish.

Compared to a fishing pole, however, where the opening in the ferrule is many times larger than the diameter of the fishing line, the tendons fill the tunnels entirely. This precision fit is a marvel to observe and helps account for the slender nature of our fingers in face of their incredible strength and adaptability. Then why is this mechanical beauty ominously called no man's land?

When a tendon gets cut, the reel is no longer connected to the fish, so to speak, and loss of finger motion is immediately evident. The good news is that surgeons can sew tendons back together, and following three months of limited activity and rehabilitation, most tendons heal with restoration of nearly normal function. That is, provided that the tendon ends have healed securely to each other but have not healed to the surrounding tissues, which would be analogous to gluing a break in the fishing line back together and at the same time gluing the repaired line to the pole.

The only way we have to keep a tendon repair site from gluing itself to the surrounding tissues is to gently glide the tendon back and forth during the healing. Gently enough so that the tendon ends do not separate, but extensive enough that the repair site does not scar to the surrounding tissues. This is the problem in no man's land.

Strong suture repairs are bulky, and prevent the tendons from gliding through the tunnels. Low-profile suture repairs are weak, and will rupture before the tendon heals. Failure occurs either way. Bunnell recognized the dilemma and advised his professional progeny against even attempting to suture tendon lacerations in this anatomically unforgiving area—no man's land. Instead, he recommended a more complicated procedure using a tendon borrowed from elsewhere in the body to bypass the injury in no man's land.

Having been told it was impossible, subsequent generations of surgeons naturally started and continue to develop ever more specialized suturing techniques that simultaneously offer stronger *and* lower-profile repairs for tendons cut in no man's land. These techniques, followed by months of carefully orchestrated hand therapy, offer hope for recovery of useful even if not always complete motion.

A moment of joy for hand surgeons is seeing their just-completed tendon repairs in no man's land glide smoothly in and out of the mouths of the narrow tunnels. An even greater joy comes when the patient has finally completed the rehab protocol and can demonstrate all the motions of the hand in their full beauty.

CHAPTER

$\overline{\quad\quad\quad\left(9\right)\quad\quad\quad}$

Artistic

HANDS

H OW WELL I REMEMBER DONNING MY FATHER'S OLD dress shirt and having my second-grade teacher spread out a big sheet of wet, glossy paper over the newspaper-protected worktable. I enjoyed the ensuing sensual, manual experience if not the final, finger-painted masterpieces. On other days, the class trundled down the hall to the music room where each of us got a set of tiny cymbals, wooden dowels, tambourines, or sandpaper blocks for "Rhythm Band." Unknown to me at the time, both activities were recapitulating the entire human experience of self-expression by creating art with our hands.

It started with our Stone Age ancestors portraying bison, horses, and deer on the walls of their caves, along with silhouettes and prints of their own hands. Thirty thousand years later, the fascination continues. For all artists, hands are tools. For some artists, hands are subjects, and in case you haven't tried, drawing a credible hand is hard. Portrait artists know this and charge considerably more if a sitter wants their hands as well as their face captured on canvas. Let's have a look at hands in art.

HANDS, PAINTED AND CARVED

Before getting started, understand that I am neither an artist nor an art historian; but being interested in hands, I like to celebrate them. Artists have created some amazing representations of the human hand over the history of civilization, and some milestones deserve recognition. So I hope to heighten your appreciation of hands and cause you to look closely the next time you view art.

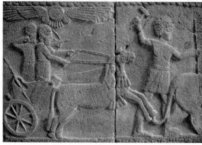

About 6000 years ago when these aforementioned southern European cave dwellers scrubbed the dust off their hands and moved to Mesopotamia, they established the first literate societies. Their drawings included lion hunts and fierce battles. Perhaps unconsciously, they depicted for the first time the power of hands affecting their lives--flinging arrows and wielding tools.

Over the next several millennia, every vertical surface in Egyptian tombs and temples seemingly became the easel for artists who mastered portrayal of the hand's grace and beauty. These sinuous, delicate fingers at work and play demonstrate the sophistication of this early yet advanced civilization. The Greeks continued this tradition of documenting the hand's participation in all aspects of life, but now on vases rather than on walls. (This made it far easier for subsequent civilizations to haul the artwork home.) Hands became part of the system of Western art. These sensual images of pouring wine, strumming stringed instruments, blessing, and caressing marked the beginning of the modern artistic era.

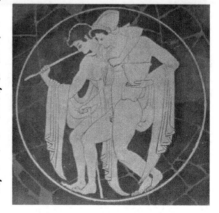

Medieval Christian painters added spiritual connotations to the hand in art—thin, even emaciated bodies exude holy awe as the hands symbolize hope and faith. Fingers bend for benedictions and blessings, plead for mercy, and cover eyes horrified by the crucifixion. Religious symbolism, not accurate anatomical representation, was the goal. These artists reserved perfection for heaven.

The Renaissance, however, changed that. Now the influence of the church waned in many spheres—religious, political, and cultural; but of paramount importance to the hand in art, the religious restrictions on human dissection dissolved. Surreptitiously at first, Michelangelo, Leonardo da Vinci, and their contemporaries discovered the mysterious structures beneath the skin that give form to the powerfully evocative hand. Not only does the hand in art now look real, it twists and turns into myriads of postures as it beholds the Christ child, steadies the heads of sages, rests on the laps of kings, and accentuates the charms of beautiful women.

Two Renaissance paintings stand out as icons of Western culture regarding hands. The first is the fresco Michelangelo painted upside down on the Sistine Chapel's ceiling. God reaches down with index 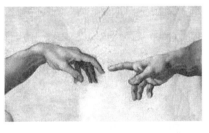 finger extended. Adam accepts the life-giving touch with grace and submission. The second, done several decades earlier, is 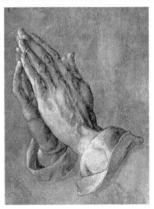 Albrecht Durer's pen and ink drawing, *Praying Hands*. Equally lifelike when compared to Michelangelo's depictions, Durer's work is revolutionary in two ways. First, the hands are old, gnarled, and by no means idealized. Second, the hands *are* the painting, not just part of it. No longer bound by the ideal, first El Greco, then Rembrandt, and later Goya allowed the hand to escape from stark reality into murky and emotional mixes of light and dark. The Impressionists also emphasized the interplay of light, but they generally depicted hands, not as lead players in their compositions, but as guides to the eye, leading the viewer to the central drama of their sun-dappled or candle-lit realms. Van Gogh, however, shunned this romantic vision and portrayed the hand of the everyday life—frugal, hardworking, and faithful.

Picasso did it all. In various moods, he depicted fingers as witty loops, bloated and stubby, stretched and foreboding, or remarkably lifelike and loving.

Artists, of course, use their own hands when they draw and paint hands. Escher playfully acknowledges this 30,000-year experience in his depiction of two hands, which are mirror images of each other and which are completing the drawing of the opposite one. In later life, Renoir was so crippled from rheumatoid arthritis that the only way he could paint was with a brush strapped to his wrist, which accounts for the broad strokes and less detail in his final style.

If we turn from two-dimensional renditions of hands to sculpture, two names stand out, Rodin and Michelangelo.

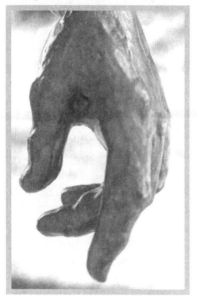

Acutely aware of the vastly expressive nature of the human hand, Rodin made hundreds of tiny clay models to capture the essence of their fluid nature and emotional power. These he kept in drawers in his studio, attaching them temporarily to his full body sculptures-in-progress to test the effect of posture and angle on the overall composition. He also used hands in isolation as subjects themselves, and although not the first to do so, he elevated such sculptures to authentic art works in their own right.

Despite this great and amazing history of the hand's depiction in art, to my mind, Michelangelo is in a league of his own. Consider the power and tension expressed in the hand of David, or the soulful, pitiful sadness conveyed by Mary's hands in the Pieta. Then consider that Michelangelo carried off this genius in marble—an awesomely unforgiving medium compared to oil or clay, truly worthy of celebration.

ART ON HANDS AND HANDS IN SAND

Two artists come to mind who have taken painting on hands to the level of a refined art form. Mario Mariotti contorted hands into various positions and then colorfully painted them, sometimes with a tiny face painted on a fingernail, to humorously represent pianists, soccer players, and weight lifters for example. Guido Daniele positions hands and fists just so and then carefully paints them to represent a myriad of amazingly lifelike animals. Google

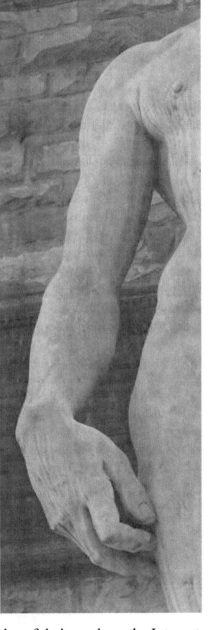

these artists' names to see examples of their work on the Internet.

Equally fascinating are videos of artists drawing with sand on backlit glass tables. It is worth a trip to YouTube to see the

149

drawings emerge, morph, and disappear while the shadowy hands above the "canvas" choreograph the display. Type in "sand art."

HAND PHOTOGRAPHY

New Yorker Henry Buhl started in investments, turned to photography, and then took to collecting seminal photographs of hands. His collection of over 1000 hand photographs reveals the entire history of photography and represents scientific, journalistic, and fine-art hands with an emphasis on contemporary art. The Guggenheim Museum exhibited 170 photographs from his collection in 2003, and highlights from this exhibit are available at www.guggenheim.org/exhibitions/buhl/highlights.html. From time to time, other museums exhibit selections from his collection. It is worth a visit. Buhl has also founded several non-profit organizations to provide job training for the homeless. One of the fundraisers is the annual sale of a calendar book that portrays a different hand photograph and a quotation about hands every week. Order it through www.ace4homeless.org.

MUSEUM HANDS

Do you have museum hands? No, I'm not talking about relics that belong in a museum but hands that feel a little puffy, stiff, and achy after leaving them relatively motionless at your sides for an hour or so—like when you visit a museum. Rings might even feel tight at such times. What's happening?

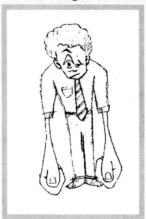

Water flows downhill. That's obvious in a river or a shower but maybe less so in our bodies, where the cellular structure simulates the composition of a sponge. Stand a moist kitchen sponge on edge for a while and note that the top edge dries out and the bottom edge gets soggy. Water flows downhill unless a pump moves it up. The heart is quite efficient at sending blood out to all parts of the body, but not so efficient at returning it. Muscle activity in our arms and legs provides auxiliary pumping for the return trip. Hence, for the feet, walking is good. Sitting still for long periods, such as on an airplane, invites the feet to swell. They become the soggy end of the sponge.

The same holds true for our hands when they hang by our sides. We do not get museum hands while we are walking briskly or shopping because our hands' and forearms' muscle activity moves that extra fluid along. The most efficient way to avoid museum hands is to hold them over your head. They then become the dry end of the sponge, but they also make you look like a hold-up victim. So to keep your hands feeling fine on your next museum visit, alternate between tight fists and wide open-finger stretches, quietly playing with your keys, or vigorously holding hands with your companion.

Any fracture, sprains, bruise, or cut greatly accentuates the soggy sponge phenomenon. The injured tissues release fluid, get stretched, and hurt. Tight rings, watchbands, or bandages can add further fluid buildup at the injury site—more swelling and more pain. Because moving the injured part hurts even more, using local muscle activity to reduce swelling is out of the question. Here, the key to comfort is elevation. Get the injured part higher than the heart and the edema fluid will flow downhill, away from the injury. Resting the injured hand on the opposite shoulder is a socially graceful option; and when nobody is judging your appearance, get that hand even higher. Resting the forearm on top of the head keeps the hand elevated and gives the head something to do. For lying down, arrange pillows to maintain the hand in a higher-than-heart position.

What about a sling? For injured hands and wrists, it is not a good idea for three reasons. A sling prevents full elevation of the hand, which enforces a museum hand and intensifies the swelling and pain. The sling substitutes for shoulder and elbow muscles when they should be contracting and pumping blood away from the injured area. Hanging a substantial and unaccustomed weight around the neck makes it ache, adding to the misery. Museum hand is bad enough. Sling neck is worse. Hands up!

FINGER PAINTING

Zhang Zao in the 8th century was the first painter to leave the brush behind. Dutch painter Cornelius Ketel (1548-1618) dabbled with the technique, and a Swiss artist, Louis Souter (1871-1942), painted at least 200 works with his fingers late in his career. Virginian Mary Ann Brandt (1921-2007) painted solely with her fingers throughout her professional career, and Arnulf Ranier (1929-) is a contemporary Austrian artist who has abstract works titled "Finger Smear" and "Hand Paintings." The handiwork of both of these contemporary artists can be viewed through Google.

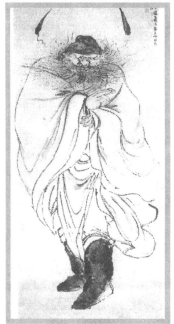

The master of finger painting, however, is Gao Quipei (pronounced Gao Chipei) (1660-1734). Gao grew up in a region remote from the major centers of artistic activity in China. As a young man he became depressed because he did not have a distinctive style of painting. His inspiration finally came to him in a dream. He began to use his fingertips and palm to apply washes and broad strokes and to use long fingernails, split like pens, to paint lines. Once certain of his style, he gave up brushes completely.

Gao's day job was in government service and he eventually became Vice Minister of Justice. This left him only several days a month to paint; but working quickly and for long hours, his lifetime production of finger paintings exceeded 50,000. Gao took advantage of his nails' fragility, completing finely detailed flowers and birds early in the day and moving on to landscapes that required broad strokes as the nails dulled and wore away. Many of his works still exist in collections around the world. The one depicted is "Zhong Kui, The Demon Queller," 1728 Liaoning Provincial Museum, Shenyang, The People's Republic of China.

An unusual technique such as finger painting does not by itself make for an important painting, but Gao's expressiveness, spontaneity, and vigor set him apart. His style influenced brush painters and stimulated others to discard the brush. Smock anyone?

I CAN QUIT ANYTIME I WANT

My wife enjoys antiques and has several collections, which she adds to particularly when we travel. The antique stores I like best have chairs by the door where those less interested can feign patience while their significant others meander seemingly forever. One day, however, she unwittingly released a monster—she bought an antique ceramic hand . . . for me. Now, the chair by the door is for her while I scrutinize every dark corner to add to my collection of several hundred glass and ceramic hands. (Yes, they also come in metal, plastic, stone, and wood, but one *must* maintain sensibility!) And since hands are the world's best tools, the ones I collect usually go beyond mere aesthetics and are crafted to hold something—coins, rings, flowers, tea, salt, cigarette ashes, candles, even whiskey and after-shave lotion (different bottles).

Moche pottery is among the most varied in the world, so it should not be surprising that this Peruvian civilization from about 400 A.D. would provide the oldest hand in my collection. It is a man's hand in terra cotta, palm down and forearm open. Sea lions cavorting in the waves are painted around the wrist.

My next oldest treasures stem from Victorian times when sentimentality reigned. Hands symbolized friendship and trust, so what could be nicer than a hand vase? Although many of these open containers are feminine hands delicately holding Grecian urns, sea

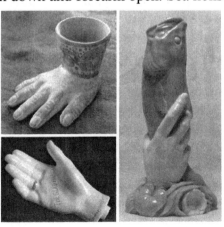

shells, or lotus flowers, my favorite is a hand rising from water lilies holding a catfish. Another, which appeals to my midwestern origins, holds an ear of corn.

Prohibition spawned "glad hands," which were conveniently corked either at the wrist or fingertip and traveled discreetly in pockets and purses. Other closed-container hands hold coins, tea, or salt and pepper.

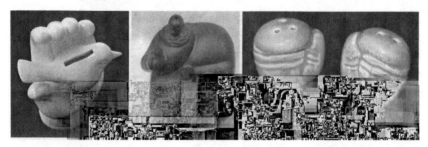

Then there are hands without openings. They merely hold. With upraised fingers they prevent wet, slippery rings from diving down the drain. With open palms they organize buttons, paperclips, loose change. And speaking of loose change, can you spare any? It's been hours since I searched eBay.

GIANT HAND SCULPTURES

For the jaded world traveler, especially one interested in hands and art, plan your next trip around visiting giant hand sculptures. To be included in my worldwide travel guide, the sculpture has to solely or principally represent hand(s) or digit(s) that are many times life-sized. It also has to be outside in a public place and not promoting a business.

The largest one is 60 feet tall. The oldest dates from Roman times. Looking for themes, a few have religious or educational connotations. Many have digits seemly emerging from the soil, and one of these is appropriately titled *The Awakening*. Some seem to beg for the viewer to recline in the comfort of the palm. Most of them, however, are just hands, sometimes reaching, which makes a giant statement regarding their importance to the sculptors. For any readers who like ears, toes, or other generally exposed body parts more than hands, I challenge them to compile a list of giant sculptures of *your* favorite part that comes anywhere near this global celebration of hands.

Many are in the centers of major cities. Others are in natural settings such as a remote South American desert. Every continent save Antarctica is represented. Botero, Cesar, and Moore are among the widely recognized sculptors. One anonymous chain-saw sculptor in Cambridge, Massachusetts, artfully sculpted a street-side tree. I have included photographs of that one and several others. Before you set off with your camera, let me warn you that these giant hands are hard to photograph. They are often on high pedestals, which means you are shooting toward a bright sky and underexposing the hand. If you get a good shot, I would enjoy seeing it.

UNITED STATES
California
Chico: Chico Municipal Center; vertical hands arching over sidewalk; painted

Fullerton: sculpture garden on Chapman Avenue; fingers cupped, palm up; stone

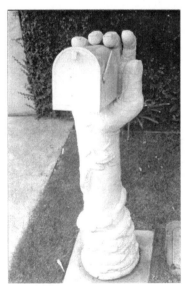

Los Angeles: Angelo Drive; hand clasping mailbox; critters on forearm; painted metal

Sacramento: Plaza 555 on Capitol Mall; two hands shaking; stone

Santa Rosa: Santa Rosa Plaza; hand resting on side with open palm; stone

Iowa
Cedar Rapids, 2nd Street SE; hand vertical with half closed fingers; heavy sheet metal

Kentucky
Berea: various locations; 12 vertical hands, slightly cupped; painted fiberglass

Louisville: Insight Training Group Building; forearms vertical, fingers intertwined; stone

Maryland

Silver Spring: in front of the National Oceanic and Atmospheric Administration; forearm vertical, palm horizontal, fingers spread; bronze

Massachusetts

Cambridge: residential street; forearm and hand vertical; tree trunk

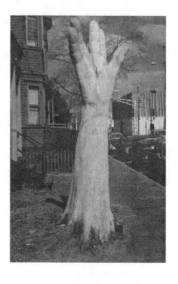

Michigan

Detroit: downtown public space; *The Fist*, tribute to Joe Louis; bronze

Missouri

Kansas City: Nelson-Atkins Museum Sculpture Park; abstract by Henry Moore; bronze

Webb City: World in Peace Memorial; praying hands; stucco over steel

New Mexico

Alamogordo: New Mexico State University; vertical forearm, hand holding diploma

New York

New York City, atop Madame Tussaud's Wax Museum; hand palm down holding rod of some sort

Oklahoma

Tulsa: Oral Roberts University; praying hands; bronze; the world's largest giant hand sculpture

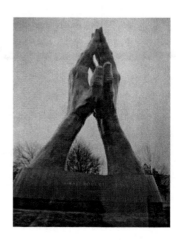

Oregon

Portland: 5th and Gilsan; vertical forearm, tips of index finger and thumb touching; bronze

Texas

Johnson City: The Benini Foundation Sculpture Ranch; two sculptures, one stone, one metal, forearms vertical, fingers straight

<u>Washington, DC</u>
Hains Point: East Potomac
 Park; hands, feet, and
 face emerging from
 ground; bronze

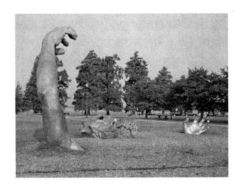

<u>AUSTRALIA</u>
Brisbane: outside a hotel;
 two separate hands, each
 with thumb and index
 fingers straight; metal
<u>BELGIUM</u>
Antwerp: City Center; hand on side with fingers extended; stone
<u>BRAZIL</u>
Sao Paulo: Memorial to Latin America; flat hand, fingers spread
 vertically; metal
<u>CANADA</u>
Quebec City: Old Quebec
 City; outstretched hand
 holding quill pen; bronze
<u>CHILE</u>
Atacama Desert: vertical
 fingers emerging from
 sand; stone
<u>CHINA</u>

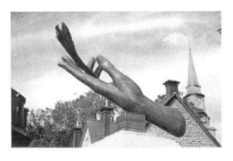

Lin Shan, near Wu Jin: hand of Buddha, fingers together; bronze
Shanghai: 6th People's Hospital; vertical hand, fingers closed,
 thumb up; stone
Hong Kong: Park Lane Shoppers Boulevard in Kowloon;
 forearms vertical, right fist clasped in left hand; bronze
<u>FRANCE</u>
Coetquidan, Brittany: Saint Cyr Military School; fisted hand
 holding flag pole
Epinal: Freedom Street; middle and ring fingers raised in victory
 sign; metal
Paris: La Defense business district; vertical thumb by Cesar;
 bright metal

Paris: Les Halles; open hand against cheek of mask; stone

Saint-Paul de Vence: Hotel l'Combre
d'Or courtyard; thumb; stone

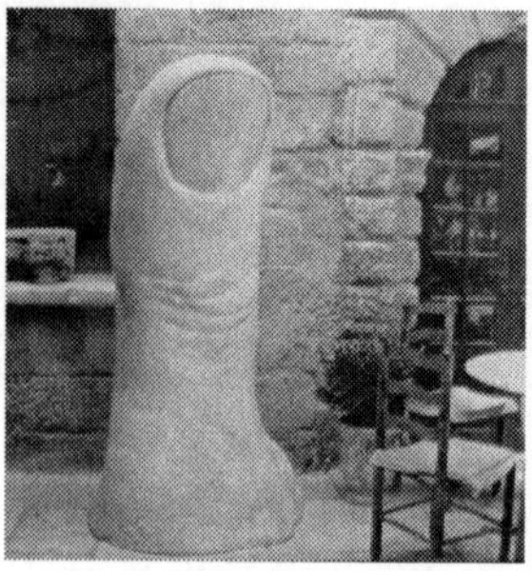

INDIA

Chandigarh: highly stylized hand with
thumb and small fingers spread away
from central fingers; metal

ISRAEL

Ramt-Gan: Shiba Hospital; stylized
vertical mitten hand; painted concrete

ITALY

Como: outside train station; two hands with widely spread
fingers; bronze

NEW ZEALAND

Wanaka, near Queensland: Roys Bay Playground; open hand on
side; metal

NIGERIA

Nsukka: University of Nigeria; open hand, palm holding kola nut

SAUDI ARABIA

Jeddah: fist; bronze

SINGAPORE

QiHua Sculpture Park; fingers rising vertically from flat surface

SOUTH AFRICA

Rustenburg, North West Province: Oude Langoed Lodge; cupped
hand; stone

SPAIN

Alicante: forearm vertical, hand holding pen; stone

Madrid: Paseo de la Castellana; vertical hand with typical Botero
distortions; bronze

SWEDEN

Eskilstuna, Stadsparken: open hand holding a small standing
person; bronze

Stockholm, next to Strombron Bridge: hand and face floating in
the water

UNITED KINGDOM

Clipstone, Nottinghamshire: Vicar Water; hand emerging from
the ground; metal

Coventry, West Midlands: Westwood Way, RSA Examination
Headquarters; hand over keyboard; stone
Dudley, West Midlands: between Wolverton Road and Southern
By-Pass; open palm facing down; cement
Edinburgh, Scotland: Leith Walk outside St. Mary's Cathedral;
horizontal hand palm up along with abstract objects; bronze
Keswick, Cumbria: hands together with palms up
Port Glasgow, Scotland: Port Glasgow High School; hand palm
up holding oil lamp
South Shields, Tyne and Wear: on bank of River Tyne; vertical
forearm and hand; bronze
Tregynon near Newtown, Wales: Gregynog Hall; vertical fingers
emerging from ground
West Bromwich, West Midlands: west end of High Street; hand
clasping cross; bronze
URUGUAY
Puente del Este: beach; fingertips emerging from sand; stone

NAZCA LINES

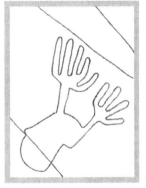

To see the world's largest hand drawings, fly several hundred miles south from
Lima, Peru, toward the city of Nazca.
Here a desert approximately 15 miles wide
and twice as long contains the doodlings
of a civilization that inhabited the area
2000 years ago. Fist-sized, reddish rocks
cover this arid, windless plateau. By
moving the rocks, the Nazcans exposed a
lighter undersurface creating lines ranging
from six inches to several hundred yards in width. The lack of
rain and dust has left their artistry undisturbed.

About 50 figures, ranging in length from 25 to 300 yards,
include whimsical renditions of a monkey, a whale, a flower, a
man, several reptiles, and 18 birds. Two hands, one with only
four digits, are attached to a strange and unidentifiable body.
More widely spread across the plateau are a series of perfectly
straight and, at times, crisscrossing lines, some running for miles.

Intermingled with these are triangles, zigzags, spirals, and other geometric shapes.

Pilots in the 1920s flying over the area discovered the Nazca lines. Archeologists disagree on how and why the terrestrially bound Nazcans made these gigantic drawings, which can be appreciated in their entirety only from above. The Nazcans aren't helping. They mysteriously disappeared after living in the area for about 500 years. For photographs and theories, google *Nazca lines*. I think the depicted Nazca figure looks like a piano player, bowler hat and all.

DID PIANISTS ASK TO HAVE THEIR TENDONS CUT?

Here is a little anatomical demonstration followed by a values question. Put your hand palm down on a flat surface as if the fingers were on a piano keyboard. Now raise your fingers one at a time off the surface. Notice how far each one lifts up. You can't lift your ring finger as high as the others, can you?

Over a hundred years ago pianists noticed this, which results from the quirky way the tendons run across the back of the hand. The tendon that raises the ring finger is tethered to the others in such a way that it has less independence. You can see this because the ring finger comes up just fine if you lift your middle finger or all your fingers at the same time.

An article in the 1887 *British Medical Journal* discusses this anatomical arrangement, which most people never even notice. The author writes, ". . . please remember that. . . [although such conditions] are minor only to our eyes and in a pathological sense; they are often of maximum importance to the sufferer, who possibly sees his livelihood in jeopardy, because his hand has forgotten its cunning." The author goes on to report that this tendon has been surgically released from its surrounding tethers both in America and in Britain, "and it is said with good results."

Hand surgeons are well aware of the ring finger's lack of independence and have all heard about this Victorian-era alteration of normal anatomy for the sake of improving keyboard "cunning." To my knowledge, however, no actual reports of the technique or the results exist, making me wonder where facts stopped and idle talk began. Would you have an operation to make your hand better than normal? What risk would you accept of the operation leaving your hand less than normal? For many, more practice might well suffice.

HOW MUCH DO MUSICIANS PRACTICE?

I occasionally see young, determined music students who come to the office because of aching muscles and sore joints. They think that if four hours of daily practice makes them good, then eight hours will make them great. After a few weeks of this intensity, their hands are in pain, clumsy, and possibly numb. Just getting dressed becomes a burden. Distraught, they want a quick fix so they can continue their ascent to Carnegie Hall. As I explain overuse syndrome, I can see disappointment spread across their faces.

Even the simplest finger motion repeated enough times and with enough force finally fatigues the tissues. Keep on doing that action, and the body aches over a wider area and for progressively longer periods after each insult. Stopping the abusive activity for a few weeks or even months usually but not always restores health to the tissues. Hence, avoidance of overuse syndrome is better than treatment.

Subtle anatomical and physiological differences among individuals may allow one to drum or strum all night and feel great, while for others, the same level of activity would be career ending. In order to inform my musician patients better, I recently posed a question on a number of philharmonic and conservatory websites. "How much do serious musicians practice?"

Most opinions were in the two- to five-hour a day range for aspiring virtuosos. Generally, mature professionals indicated that they practice less. The thread that ran through all the responses, however, was to practice smart, not hard. Their summarized advice seems useful even for amateurs.

1. Use an appropriately sized and well-maintained instrument, Otherwise, it demands more work.
2. Always warm up. This is an athletic endeavor. A cold start invites injury.

3. Take frequent breaks to relax and stretch. Two or three short practice sessions a day are better than one long one.

4. Critique your technique. Avoid postures that require constantly tensed muscles. Find postures that keep wrist and finger joints out of extreme positions. Use the minimal force to achieve the desired effect. Practicing with bad habits or bad form is worse than not practicing.

5. Repetition alone will not solve a technical problem. Experiment with different fingering or different finger and wrist postures until the passage flows smoothly.

6. Know your limits. Your friends and teachers may be able to play in three ensembles and practice for hours. You may not.

7. Consider the impact of other activities that may be pushing you toward overuse, for example computer, video games, sports.

8. Pain is a sign that you are doing something wrong. Do not ignore it. Slow down.

9. Rest, anti-inflammatory medication, stretching, and careful strengthening may help, so seek medical attention, but cautiously. If the doctor recommends an operation, get another opinion. Surgery rarely helps.

Does the last recommendation surprise you? Not me. Think of it like this. Musicians get paid because they can perform at, say, 103% of normal human capacity. When they drop to 101% of human capacity, they are distraught. An operation never restores complete normalcy. There is always scarring. Surgery works when it can take hands functioning at 20%-70% of normal capacity and increase their function to 95%. Operating on a hand functioning at 101% of normal capacity is going to make it worse, not better.

LEGENDARY MUSICAL HANDS

Sergey Rachmaninov was one of the greatest pianists of the 20th century. He also conducted and composed with great skill. His compositions, however, are notoriously hard to play because he wrote large chords for his own extraordinarily large hands. His long fingers were said to cover the keyboard like octopus tentacles. For example, Rachmaninov could span an octave and a half and could play a chord such as C, E^b, G, C, and G easily with his left hand. That requires a span of about 12 inches. Even more amazing, with his right hand he would play a chord such as C (index finger), E, G, C (small finger), and then reach under with his thumb and play the next higher E! Rachmaninov was reserved, unsmiling, even grave, and although his fingers performed with passion, his face and body remained still and seemingly uninvolved.

Contrast Rachmaninov's demeanor to that of another legendary musician from a century before. This man became the "incarnation of desire, scorn, madness, and burning pain" through the medium of his violin, which he apparently never practiced and which he pawned from time to time to pay gambling debts. He reveled in the nocturnal vices, at least until he contacted syphilis. The large doses of mercury taken for treatment account for the early loss of his teeth and development of a "corpse-like" complexion. "Excessive nervousness," "irritable bowel," and a probable diagnosis of tuberculosis also contributed to his wasted appearance, further accentuated by baggy clothes. Yet concertgoers by the hundreds thronged after Nicolo Paganini in the streets to get a glimpse of the "King of Violinists," the "Demon of Fiddlers," the "Virtuoso in Excelsis." Stories abound regarding his ability to play the most difficult passages with speed, clarity, intonation, and expressivity--on untuned strings or with two or even three strings missing.

Paganini's hands contributed to this level of showmanship not seen before or since. Contrasted to Rachmaninov's, Paganini's hands were actually smaller than average, but physicians who examined them remarked that they moved as if they were without muscles or bones. His finger joints were said to move from side to side with equal facility as that with which they opened and closed. As a party trick, Paganini would effortlessly bend his thumb backwards until its nail touched the back of his hand. This extreme flexibility allowed him to position his fingers in seemingly impossible positions on the strings, for instance to play C's on all four strings simultaneously. This requires a reach of more than six inches between the index and small fingers, which is an astounding feat when the fingers are curled around the violin neck.

Physicians speculate as to whether Rachmaninov and Paganini both had genetic conditions to account for their remarkable hands. If so, they both certainly put them to good use.

WAVING HANDS

Through an orchestral conductor's manual gestures come some of the most emotionally evocative sensations possible. The work can be strenuous without even a measure's rest for pieces of symphonic length. Even so, this highly visible endeavor purportedly gives conductors longer life than any other occupation. How do a conductor's hands transform printed squiggles into high art?

Some music could be played passably well without a conductor if the players could agree on a starting point, a tempo, and an interpretation and if they could continuously hear one another. Agreement among musicians, however, is no more likely than agreement among politicians; and even though musicians listen carefully, they cannot hear the composite sound. Enter the magician, wand and all.

The conductor selects the program and carefully studies, if not memorizes, the scores. Then through love or fear, he gains the orchestra's attention, if not respect, and imparts his interpretation on the composition. His gestures convert an age-old system of dots on lines into reality.

It is a universally recognized sign language. A conductor can make a guest appearance anywhere in the world, and regardless of spoken-language barriers, his manual interpretation can readily convert the notations into awe-inspiring sound.

Unseen by the audience, facial gestures embellish the conductor's manual signs, and body language adds style. Some conductors are frugal with their movements, while others are quite animated and flamboyant. Regardless, conductors are taught to relax. They shun jerky hand movements and rigid postures in order to avoid an identical tension in the music.

Dance instruction often improves a novice conductor's gracefulness and fluidity.

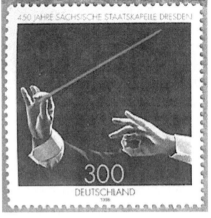

The baton is a highly visible extension of the conductor's right forearm, and this keeps the rhythm. The left hand is free to draw out nuances such as crescendo, vibrato, and phrasing. As the conductor turns to look from one section to another, he must remember to keep both hands visible to the entire orchestra. It may sound easy, but consider patting your head in syncopated staccato and rubbing your stomach in 5/4 time. All the while discerning patrons are staring at your collar and 100 musicians, many of whom want your job, engulf you with sound. Eugene Ormandy described the job this way:

> He must be prepared to instantaneously make any adjustments, large or small, in the actual performance required for the fullest realization of his inner concept. Many factors make this necessary: a different hall, a player's momentary inattention, the effect of several thousand persons upon the acoustics, even the understandable enthusiasm of performance, which might affect the tempo. At such a moment the conductor meets his greatest challenge, for the progress of the work must not suffer in the slightest; there must be no detectable "hitch." At such moments the experience of a conductor tells, for the young conductor, new to such emergencies, tends to one thing at a time. Music does not permit this, for it flows in time, and all adjustments must be superimposed upon the uninterrupted continuum.

All with the mere wave of a hand.

APPLAUSE

It seems so natural to slap our hands together. Seals do it. Babies do it. We clap to get somebody's attention, to keep time to music, and especially to sound approval.

Have you ever been part of an audience where the initial chaotic thunder spontaneously became synchronized clapping? A moment later the applause may go chaotic and then again rhythmic—a unified appreciation. Several physicists wanted to know why these waves of synchronized clapping occur. They placed microphones in concert halls and measured the intensity and speed of clapping from the entire audience as well as from individual concertgoers who were unaware of the test.

After an initial bout of rapid, chaotic clapping, the audience instinctively begins to slow down and to clap in time with those around them. The sound of each collective clap is, of course, quite loud and demonstrative. The time between individual claps, however, is nearly doubled, so the overall sound level goes down. This drop in volume compels the audience to clap faster, but individuals have different speeds of fast clapping, and the synchronization is broken.

The finale is a website where the hands by themselves actually make music rather than merely express appreciation. If you cup your hands together and squeeze the air out between your fingers, small squeaks may occur. Can you imagine turning those squeaks into recognizable music and making money from it? It is called manualism. For a trek to the edge, go to www.handman.com.

Walt Whitman:
> O to have life henceforth
> a poem of new joys!
> to dance, clap hands…

IN A MANNER INCAPABLE OF IMITATION

If you are still not convinced that hands are an integral part of the arts, both performing and participatory, consider this. What if dancers kept their hands in their pockets? To begin with, both waltzing cheek to cheek and swinging your square-dance or jitterbug partner would be problematic. And without hands, I suspect that the chicken dance, the Macarena, Y.M.C.A., and the Hokey Pokey would have all fallen off the charts long ago. For no other reason, those of us who are coordination-challenged find that holding our arms out helps with our balance.

So as long as the arms are flailing around, the hands might as well add to the joy by clapping or even by taking up castanets or finger cymbals. Good dancers, of course, can greatly add to the poise and beauty of a dance with graceful arm and finger movements. I marvel at the ballerina who, seriously out of breath and standing on the ends of her big toes, continues to smile and remembers to arc her fingers gracefully to add every possible embellishment to the performance.

Dancing hands can also tell stories. In India, traditional dancers study and perfectly duplicate 32 major hand positions, 24 combined hand positions, and 12 movements. By combining these elements and adding minor variations, the possibilities for symbolic gesturing are nearly limitless. These gestures originated in Buddhism, and their meanings expanded and changed as they spread through Asia. A Chinese dance troupe has gained world-wide fame for their performances of the Thousand Hand Bodhisattva Dance. Take a quick break and google "thousand hand dance" to see a short video clip. Then because they are next, google "hula gestures." A PBS website should be at the top of the list. Watch the graceful Hawaiian dance gestures and then come right back.

An interesting question, raised by an anthropologist, is whether the symbolic gestures from Indian dance found their way into Indonesia and then across the Pacific in ancient times to influence the hula. In both, the production of gestures is identical. The movement flows out from the shoulder to the hand and ends in the gracefully positioned fingers. There are far fewer gestures for Hawaiian dance than there are for Indian dance, but some are identical. For instance, keeping the fingers straight while touching all their tips together symbolizes *flower bud* in India and *flower* in Hawaii. When the dancer makes this gesture near the mouth, it means *speech* in India and *talk* or *song* in Hawaii. The gestures for house, fish, rain, and half moon are also identical, which could just be coincidental, resulting from the hands imitating the object they are representing. But both cultures also have identical dance gestures for abstract concepts such as death (downward movement of the hands) and unity or marriage (fingers intertwined).

One thing that is certain, however, is that the hula hip movements are different than in Hindu dances. In 1933, an Australian on observing the hula wrote, ". . . the effect was most striking as the dancers moved around the circle, stopping frequently to rotate the hips and wriggle the legs in a manner incapable of imitation by a European." I am not sure if he even noticed the graceful and highly symbolic hand gestures.

CHAPTER

(10)

HANDS

In Popular Culture

THE IROQUOIS INDIANS ATTRIBUTE THE GEOGRAPHY OF central New York State to the Great Spirit, who is said to have blessed the land with the imprint of his hands. Indeed, a series of nearly parallel, finger-like lakes nestle between previously glacier-covered ridges. The rolling country-side has been prime agricultural land since the time of the Indians. Today vineyards, orchards, and dairy farms share the hills with dense forest. From west to east the lakes are gracefully named Conesus, Hemlock, Candice, Honeoye, Canandaigua, Keuka, Seneca, Cayuga, Owasco, Skaneateles, and Otisco, and collectively are, of course, known as the Finger Lakes. Yes, there are eleven, but when Indians roamed this area, they may have been enjoying the scenery rather than carefully counting.

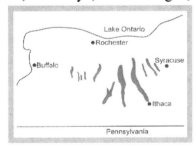

Hands, fingers, and even thumbs have permeated their way into nearly every crevice of popular culture: expressions, songs, movie plots, and place names to cite a few. Let's start with thumbs.

THE THUMB IN POPULAR CULTURE

Tom Thumb is a miniature rose. Tom Thumb is a Pomeranian breed of tiny dogs. Typewriters and archery bows designed for children and a miniature golf course are called Tom Thumb. Who is this guy?

You may have heard of General Tom Thumb; he was a 19th century sensation—made so by P.T. Barnum. He was born Charles Stratton, tall enough as an adult to barely see across a kitchen counter. Barnum took him in as a child, renamed him, and trained him to sing, dance, and imitate famous people. They toured the world and met many heads of state, including Lincoln. Always suave with the women, Tom married Lavinia Bump, who was eye level with a desktop. Their wedding was one of the most important social events in New York City that winter. The newlyweds greeted their 2000 reception guests while standing on a grand piano. Tom and Lavinia later departed on a three-year world tour, appearing over 1400 times in nearly 600 cities. That is not a small feat.

Even before Stratton appeared, a steam engine promoter built a small locomotive and named it, surprise, Tom Thumb. In a famous race the owner pitted the little iron horse against a big stagecoach steed. The locomotive was leading until an engine belt slipped. The horse won, but we remember Tom Thumb.

A hundred years before the horse race, the little guy shows up in a London play, *The Tragedy of Tragedies: or The Life and Death of Tom Thumb the Great.* He makes his debut in a book a hundred years before that, *History of Tom Thumbe, the Little, for his small stature surnamed, King Arthurs Dwarfe: Whose Life and adventures, containe many strange and wonderful accidents, published for the merry time-spenders.*

Ancient oral legend has it that a ploughman's wife wished for a son even if he were no bigger than her husband's thumb. Merlin grants the wish. Various folktales recount Tom's noble deeds as King Arthur's smallest knight. He was also a giant slayer and a ladies' man. In one version Tom dies from a spider's poisonous breath.

So look at your thumb and imagine a gallant knight standing there. Imagine the possibilities. May the lighthearted saga for merry time-spenders continue, sponsored by your hand.

Compared to Tom Thumb, Thumbelina has a straightforward lineage. She arose from Hans Christian Andersen's pen. A woman planted a special barleycorn that she purchased from a fairy. The seed sprouted and turned into a tulip, which, when the woman kissed it, opened up to reveal a delicate, graceful maiden, scarcely half as long as a thumb.

Though often retold in books and movies, the tale was a children's story from the first and has remained essentially unchanged. Thumbelina's charm and good heart overcome multiple adversities and ultimately bring her to the delicately winged flower prince. Every flower contains a beautiful tiny man and woman, he explains. The prince asks Thumbelina to be his wife and renames the new queen Maia. Varieties of miniature zinnias, hostas, and carrots are named Thumbelina. Look for the royal couple in every blossom.

You can find thumbs on maps as well. West Thumb is a projection of Yellowstone Lake. From the air, it looks more like a doorknob, but it was named in 1870 from the vantage point of a canoe.

Michigan, however, is a different story. It consists of two separate land masses, each surrounded on three sides by water. With just a little imagination, the lower peninsula looks like a mitten and the blunt projection into Lake Huron is Michigan's Thumb. This five-county region is an agricultural and recreational area. I suppose that in a wet year it is the earth's largest green thumb. But if a dry year makes an economic downturn here worse than in the rest of the state, it sticks out. When you ask people from Michigan's lower peninsula where they are from, they will likely show you by pointing to their town's location on their hand.

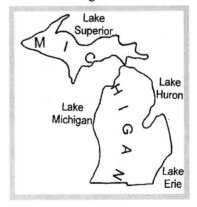

IN A MANNER OF SPEAKING

Thumbs also frequently occur as figures of speech--for instance, all thumbs, two thumbs up, thumbs down, green thumb, thumb a ride, under one's thumb, thumbnail sketch, rule of thumb, thumb through, sore thumb, thumbed, and thumb one's nose. Other parts of the hand also add color to English: white-knuckle experience, knuckle sandwich, knuckle down, fingered, light fingers, five-finger requisition, lady finger, sticky fingers, butter fingers, iron fist, palm off, and grease a palm.

Moving up the arm, anatomy-based expressions include limp wrist. sharp elbows, elbow in, elbow grease, bend an elbow, rub elbows, elbow room, strong-armed, heavily armed, armchair, arm of a lake/government, big shoulders, shoulder responsibility, shoulder the blame, and cold shoulder.

With that introduction, let's nose in on a presentation about the winner for body-based expressions.

THE COVERT MISSION

"I will hand in the final report tomorrow. For this debriefing I will hand out copies of my outline done in long hand as well as my shorthand notes, both of which refer to the handbook. I know your hands are full, but keep it handy for future reference because the manual demonstrates first hand the hand of the master. Shall we start?

"Despite the hand-in-glove planning, at the last minute the hand-picked boarding party could not locate the critical handmade handle. Their hands were tied and the mission stalled, but following an offhand suggestion, they signaled headquarters. A replacement was on hand here, and in several hours the boarding party had it in hand.

"On one hand that delay appeared costly, but on the other hand, it allowed the raid to proceed in total darkness. Professionals that they are, they played the hand they were dealt, and our team finally floated alongside the yacht. The former ranch hand, now disguised as a handyman in secondhand clothes, positioned himself, opened his toolbox, and handled the handle with care. He weighed its heft and gave it an experienced overhand throw. The rope ladder was secure.

"Climbing hand over hand, all four quickly reached the deck. After brief hand-to-hand fighting, Juan single-handedly subdued the guard, who was dressed shabbily in hand-me-downs and was said to be caught dreaming of a hand-in-hand walk with his lover, but that was third-hand information. The gamblers and bookmakers in the galley slowly responded to the clatter and to the guard's muffled shouts for all hands on deck. They quickly fell into enemy hands—well, ours. After other commands went unheeded, "Hands up!" proved to be the hands down way to get the bookies to hand over their notes.

"Our heavy-handed handler treated the captives evenhandedly by placing them all in handcuffs. He smirked that it would be unwise for any of them to try their hand at escape. Before he could hand on other advice, Allisha rolled onto the deck in her wheelchair and ordered that the command be handed off to her. (A captive later told me that she had glad-handed her way on board earlier in the day, offered them favors, but then proved quite a handful while covering for the team's delay.) We had given her a free hand, and now Allisha exerted her iron hand, wrapped the handgun that had been handed over into a handwoven handkerchief, and stuffed it in her handbag along with a handball that was loose on the deck. Hissing that that she was nobody's handmaiden, she asked for a helping hand with the rest of the cleanup. No one, however, lent a hand, although the humiliated guards gave her a hand when she finished.

"Then Allisha, an old hand at bookmaking, focused on the issue at hand, faced our ham-handed competitors, and grimly handed down the edict. Only handicapped handicappers could handpick bets in all future events, even simple handcart races. Those underhanded bookies, caught red-handed, would have to keep their hands off our hands-on operation, although for most that would mean begging for handouts with hat in hand, working as hired hands, or possibly even going empty-handed. They reluctantly nodded their agreement, recognizing that control was permanently out of their hands. One mumbled that he was washing his hands of the entire business and gave Allisha a backhanded compliment for her role in his career change.

"We really have to hand it to the team for a job well done. May I see a show of hands for approving the report?"

(Of course the covert mission was actually to use as many different "hand" expressions (81) in a quasi-coherent story of minimal length (600 words). Do you want to try your hand?)

FAMOUS HANDPRINTS

Grauman's Chinese Theater in Hollywood must be the most famous movie theater in the world. Since its opening in 1927, over 200 actors and actresses have made lasting impressions in its Forecourt of the Stars. All have signed their names in sections of cement pavement. Many have left shoe prints. Shirley Temple stood barefoot. Betty Grable pressed a leg into action. Jimmy Durante printed his schnoz. George Burns included a cigar. Some big, some small, one fist—nearly all made images of their hands. I wonder why that is?

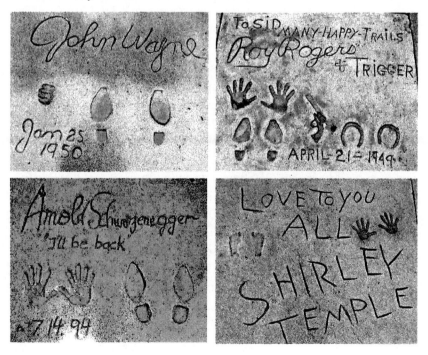

I KNOW IT LIKE THE BACK OF MY HAND

People use the above statement to imply that they know something really well. Is it a fair measure? How well do we really know the backs of our hands? Without looking at your hands, try answering these five questions that a researcher asked 60 people.

1. Does your index finger have hair over the back of its middle segment?
2. Is your ring finger or your index finger longer?
3. Is your thumbnail wider than it is long, or is it longer than it is wide?
4. Do you have any nonsurgical scars on your hands?
5. Is a crescent-shaped white band visible at the base of your ring-finger nail?

Now have a look at your hand. How many did you get right? Surprised? In the study, the average number of correct responses was 2.7. Women more accurately answered the first question than men. Otherwise men and women scored equally. Only one subject missed all five questions, and only one subject (a hand therapist) got all five correct. The fraction of people correctly answering each question hovered around 50%. Flipping a coin would produce the same results. In other words, at least for these questions, we are not entirely familiar with the backs of our hands and should be wary of those who claim they are. Other claims may be as spurious.

THROWING HANDS IN ANTWERP AND ULSTER

Antwerp is Belgium's second largest city. The birthplace of Peter Paul Rubens, it started as a river port during Roman times and has become the world's diamond center. Local legend tells of a giant who would extract tolls from boatmen navigating the river and who cut off the hands of noncompliant travelers. A Roman legionnaire ended this nonsense by slaying the ogre and flinging his huge hand into the river. *Hantwerpen* was the spelling of the city for centuries and means throwing the hand.

Unearthing a giant skeleton years later further substantiated the legend. The local museum displayed these remains until somebody realized that they were whale bones. Scholarly research ensued and turned up *aanwerp*—soil deposited in a river delta—as the actual source of the city's name.

Undaunted by reality, the locals commemorate the brave legionnaire with a bronze sculpture in the main plaza. Hands remain on the city's coat of arms. Sweet shops sell hand-shaped cookies and chocolates. The hallmark for locally produced gold and silverware is, you guessed it, a hand.

Throwing somebody else's hand is one thing. Throwing your own is something else. Ulster, Ireland's northernmost province, has as part of its heraldic crest a red hand. Various myths surround the origin of this symbol, and this one is a good match for the Antwerp story. In an effort to inspire his troops, the leader of a force invading by ship offered the largest section of land to the warrior whose hand first touched the ground. So one of the men cut off his own hand and flung it ashore. Like it or not, these tales introduce the genre of the disembodied hand and its powers.

A GOTHIC STORY

Fearful of ridicule, British author Horace Walpole published *The Castle of Otranto* anonymously in 1764. It was an immediate success, and Walpole took credit when the second edition appeared only four months later. Innumerable subsequent editions of *Otranto* have appeared. At the time the story captivated readers owing to the "highly finished" characters of "spirit and propriety," to quote two early reviewers. Today, *The Castle of Otranto* owes its reputation to initiating a genre—the Gothic novel, which might be summed up as a soap opera in an ancient setting.

Manfred, prince of Otranto, had one son and one daughter. The latter, a most beautiful virgin, aged eighteen, was called Matilda. Conrad, the son, was three years younger, a homely youth, sickly, and of no promising disposition; yet he was the darling of his father, who never showed any symptoms of affection to Matilda.

Set in the Dark Ages, it is a tale of pride, greed, mistaken identity, Crusader chivalry, love at first sight, and torn allegiances. Manfred's ancestors usurped Otranto, and he connived to make his hold legitimate through a marriage of Conrad to the family of the rightful owners. After Conrad's sudden and mysterious death, Manfred desperately proposed himself and then Matilda as marriage partners.

When interceding monks and various supernatural omens failed to halt Manfred's chicaneries, Walpole performed another literary first—calling on a disembodied hand.

Oh! my lord, my lord! cried she, we are all undone! It is come again! It is come again!—What is come again? cried Manfred amazed.--Oh! the hand! the giant! the hand! Support me! I am terrified out of my senses, cried Bianca. . . . I saw upon the uppermost banister of the great stairs a hand in armour as big, as big—I thought I should have swooned . . .

Manfred finally saw the errors of his ways just before the world literally collapsed around him. The characters of spirit and propriety lived happily ever after. Maudlin? Definitely. A literary milestone? Yes. A subsequent need for disembodied hands in popular culture? You decide.

MOVIE HANDS

The only movies where hands play a leading role are horror movies, where, of course, the hands are disembodied and go their own way. The granddaddy of these is *The Beast with Five Fingers* (1946). Several murders occur at the estate of a pianist who fell, possibly with help, to his death. Has the pianist's severed hand returned to strangle the characters who are arguing over his will?

Others in the genre include *The Crawling Hand* (1963), *The Hand* (1981), *Summer School* (1987), *Evil Dead II* (1987), *Demonoid, Messenger of Death* (1991), and *Severed Ties* (1992). Their Internet movie reviews are salted with such descriptions as "teenage gross-out," "cheap B movie," "lame," and "unintended laughs." So if you can cite the plots of all of these and add other disembodied hand movies to the list, you might want to get outside more. Having said that, actors and directors in these movies include Peter Lorre, Michael Caine, and Oliver Stone.

If a disembodied hand can be lovable, the winner would be Thing, appearing in the TV series *The Addams Family* for several years in the 1960s and in the movie by the same title in 1991. Thing is the family pet and, when unable to communicate by gesture alone, taps out messages in Morse code. Thing distributes mail, lights cigars, answers phones, and even goes to work for FedEx when the family budget gets tight.

Even though disembodied hands have not grabbed any Oscars, the absence of hands has. *The Best Years of Our Lives*, which I mentioned in Chapter 4, won Best Picture in 1946. Three World War II veterans return to peacetime life in a small town and attempt to readjust. One of them, portraying himself, had both hands blown off in a naval explosion and displays amazing facility with bilateral hook prostheses for all daily tasks, including lighting his cigarettes with book matches. He does, however, have difficulty allowing others to accept his altered sense of self. Far beyond showing what a motivated amputee can do without real fingers, the movie is a serious, compelling drama.

For whimsy, the award goes to *Edward Scissorhands* (1990). Although the title suggests that the movie should be in the same category as those with "Demonoid" or "Severed" in their titles, this mix of fairy-tale and social satire received wide critical and box office appeal. Think of it as *Beauty and the Beast* set in suburbia. With scissors for hands, Edward is a whiz at shaping topiary and ice sculptures but struggles when fastening buttons, eating peas, and generally fitting in.

For the movie that has it all, the two-thumbs-up award goes to *The Fugitive* (1993), which, like *The Addams Family*, started out as a television series. Here, a physician is accused of murdering his wife. While evading the police, he hunts down the real culprit, who the Fugitive senses is one-handed. Drama, thrills, suspense, and action—it is all here. Popcorn anyone? Just remember that eating in the dark with scissors or hooks could be dangerous, and who knows what could be lurking underneath the seats.

MOVIES NOT REALLY ABOUT HANDS

A Farewell to Arms (1932, 1957)
The Man with the Golden Arm (1955)
The Left Hand of God (1955)
Tom Thumb (1958)
Goldfinger (1964)
Five Finger Exercise (1962)
Cool Hand Luke (1967)
I Wanna Hold Your Hand (1978)

THE ORIGINAL DISEMBODIED HAND

Synopsis: Enemy troops are raiding nearby and an attack on the empire's capital city is imminent. The city, however, is safe. Its surrounding wall is insurmountable. The wall not only embraces extensive land for growing crops, it also straddles a river. Thus, if besieged, those inside are ensured of limitless nourishment.

To show his lack of concern about the advancing enemy, the king proudly hosts a wild party for a thousand courtesans. The flow of wine and wanton revelry come to an abrupt halt, however, when a hand appears on the wall of the banquet hall and writes four words, which make no sense. The shaken king calls on his advisers and offers them purple clothes, a gold chain, and a promotion to the empire's third in command if they can interpret the handwriting on the wall. All fail, which further unnerves the king.

The queen hears the abrupt change in mood coming from the banquet hall, enters, and consoles her husband. She advises him to seek the counsel of a man who previously interpreted dreams, riddles, and other conundrums for the king's father. The man is brought before the king and is offered the same rewards that the king previously offered his regular advisers. The man waves off the reward but interprets the writing. The four words on the wall say that because of the king's hubris and worship of false idols, his kingdom is ending.

Meanwhile, the attacking army has diverted the flow of the river. The invaders walk easily along the empty riverbed, underneath the formidable wall, and into the city. Inside they kill the king and conquer the empire.

City/Empire	Babylon/Babylonia
Attackers	Persians
King	Belshazzar
Man	Daniel
Original source:	*Old Testament*, Daniel 5

A ONE-ACT, TWO-HAND PLAY

Roy: "Hey Bill, over here."
Bill: (raises hand with palm out and fingers loose, moves hand from side to side)
Roy: "How ya been?"
Bill: (firmly grasps Roy's right hand with his right hand, moves it up and down several times)
Roy: "I'm still procrastinating on writing a piece on hand gestures for my book."
Bill: (extends both index fingers, rubs the left one along the side of the right one several times)
Roy: "Yeah, I know they're important, but just making a list would be boring. I'll skip it, nobody will miss. . ."
Bill: (raises index finger, waves it from side to side)
Roy: "Well, wahshudido?"
Bill: (cups hand behind ear)
Roy: "Sorry, I was mumbling. What should I do?"
Bill: (strokes chin with thumb on one side, other fingers on the other, then taps the side of his head with his index finger)
Roy: "Okay, tell me."
Bill: (places palm on abdomen and moves it in a circle)
Roy: "Me too. Let's go eat. You can tell me over lunch. I'll buy."
Bill: (places palms together, rubs them quickly back and forth)
Roy: "Somehow, I'll have to make the piece interesting."
Bill: (fingertips bunched together pointing up, moves hand away from body a short distance)
Roy: "How's your salad?"

Bill: (spreads fingers with palm down, rotates forearm slightly back and forth)
Roy: "Mine's delicious."
Bill: (points thumb up, other fingers closed)
Roy: "Coffee?"
Bill: (touches tip of thumb to tip of index fingers, other fingers nearly straight)
Roy: "Dessert?
Bill: (holds straightened fingers together, faces palm out, moves hand from side to side)
Roy: "I think I know what I can do to describe gestures."
Bill: (places straightened fingers together and brings them to cover open mouth)
Roy: "I'll get a video camera and go around capturing examples of people gesturing on the street, at work, at the gym because gestures in one culture may mean entirely something else in another. Then I'll put them on a CD, hire a narrator, and. . ."
Bill: (holds palm out with fingers together, brings fingers down to contact thumb three times)
Roy: "A professional narrator would be best, and then I'll get. . ."
Bill: (holds one hand vertical with straightened fingers together, then brings the other flattened hand down horizontally on top of first hand)
Roy: "So what's wrong with my idea?"
Bill: (pinches nose between thumb and index finger)
Roy: "Why? "
Bill: (holds palm up with tips together, rubs thumb back and forth across other fingertips)
Roy: "Maybe I can get a loan?"
Bill: (makes small loops against side of head with straightened index finger)
Roy: "You got a better idea?"
Bill: (with palm up, moves index finger repeatedly from straight to curved position)
Roy: "Why, is somebody going to steal your idea?"
Bill: (points index finger straight up and brings it to lips)
Roy and Bill put their heads together for a minute and whisper.
Roy: "Hey, that's great. Awesome."

Bill: (cups fingers, blows on tips, and rubs them on chest)

Roy: "I've gotta get started. D'you see the waiter?"

Bill: (holds tips of thumb, index, and middle fingers together with palm down, makes squiggly motion from left to right)

Roy: "My wallet? I must have left it at home. I'm not going to be able to pay after all."

Bill: (strikes forehead with heel of hand)

Roy: "Can you take care of it and I'll pay you back?"

Bill: (crosses index and middle fingers)

Roy: "Yeah, I'm sorry. It seems like I always forget my wallet."

Bill: (with palm down and fingers straight, bumps side of index finger against eyebrows several times)

Roy: "I understand how you must feel. Really, I'm sorry."

Bill: (with palm facing body and relaxed fingers directed down, flicks hand away from body three times)

Roy: "You're a pal. I'm outta here. I'll let you proofread my paper when it's done."

Bill: a. (points index finger up with other fingers closed, makes small circles with hand)

    b. (looks at audience, turns palms up at shoulder level, raises hands several times)

    c. (brings fingertips to puckered lips, then turns palm up and blows across straightened fingers)

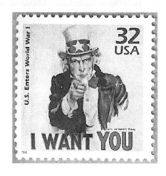

CHAPTER

$$11$$

High-Tech

HANDS

ATCHING QUIZ. WHO YA GONNA CALL?

Symptoms
1 Shoulder and arm ache while blow-drying hair
2 Whole arm aches after a 70-hour week on the computer
3 Multiple joints are swollen, hot, and painful
4 Nail bed has a dark patch
5 Hands shake involuntarily
6 Fingertips are cool and dusky
7 Wrist is stiff months after a fracture has healed

Specialist
A Thoracic surgeon
B Rehabilitation medicine specialist
C Rheumatologist
D Dermatologist
E Neurologist
F Cardiologist
G Hand therapist

So far in the book, when not just having fun, I have mostly discussed ways hand surgeons treat hands. The appendages, however, are not entities unto themselves. Diseases such as rheumatoid arthritis and stroke of course affect the hand, and treatment of these diseases requires other specialists as noted in

183

the quiz. (To make scoring easy, the correct specialists are already listed in the order that corresponds to the list of symptoms.) This chapter explores the multitude of disciplines complementing hand surgery and the high-tech innovations that have an impact on the care and treatment of the hand.

IS IT TIME FOR HAND TRANSPLANTATION?

For 40 years, surgeons have been sewing amputated parts back on the *same* person. The surgery is technically demanding, time-consuming, widely practiced, and well accepted as a medical advance.

The concept of replacing a missing or severely injured hand with a normal hand from *another* person, recently deceased, is perhaps bizarre, but appealing. Abnormal or absent digits could be similarly replaced—a sort of spare parts substitution that might well improve quality of life for the recipient. After all, the benefit of life-saving organ transplants—hearts, lungs, and livers—is well known. Is it time for hands to join the list?

Just maybe, for various reasons. Foremost is biological reality. Each of our bodies has an extremely strong immunologic sense of self. Circulating antibodies and white cells recognize foreign proteins from bacteria or cancer cells, for instance, and our immune systems make heroic efforts to eradicate such alien material. It is vital to our survival.

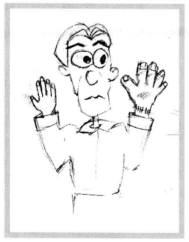

If death is impending because of a failing, vital organ such as the heart or liver, it may be worthwhile to try persuading the immune system to ignore a transplanted organ. Various potent drugs can suppress the immune system and diminish our body's sense of self. But the drugs themselves can make the hand recipient extremely sick, and they also leave him vulnerable to infection and cancer.

Most people would agree that *possible* death from infection or cancer is an acceptable risk compared to facing *certain,* early death from a failed vital organ. So heart transplant patients take immunosuppressive drugs for life and walk a narrow line. Too little medicine risks letting the immune system reject the organ. Too much medicine risks leaving the body totally defenseless against cancer cells and bacteria.

As it turns out, our immune systems have extremely strong opinions about the proteins in other people's skin and bone marrow, tissues not found in internal organs. Transplanted hands or digits, of course, would expose the recipient's immune system to both donor skin and bone marrow. These foreign proteins are going to cause an extreme reaction, suppressed only by intensive, life-long drug treatment. In this instance, most people agree that greatly risking death from cancer or from strep throat complications is unacceptable compared to living healthfully with a missing or deficient hand.

Most doctors agree that subjecting a healthy young adult to decades of life-threatening immunosuppression in turn for gaining a hand is not a fair trade. The gritty details do not make good sound bites and so get lost behind the fanfare. For people missing both hands, the medical opinion regarding hand transplantation is more nuanced.

As immunosuppressive drugs become safer and more effective, skin transplantation for burn victims and limb and partial limb transplantation for people with congenital absences or traumatic losses may become daily occurrences.

Recent experimental develop-ments may entirely change the way we look at all transplants, whether they are kidneys, hearts, livers, hands, or nearly any other part. Rather than chronically suppressing the body's immune response to prevent rejection, work is under way to briefly overwhelm the body's

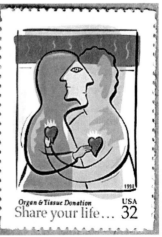

Organ & Tissue Donation USA
Share your life... 32

sense of self. When it recovers, the body will not recognize the newly transplanted tissue as foreign. This is known as tolerance in medical circles and is somewhat akin to convincing your spouse that the dent in the bumper has always been there. Consequences could still be fatal during the time the immune system is overwhelmed, but thereafter antirejection medication would be unnecessary. Easy and effective establish-ment of tolerance could revolutionize transplant surgery.

WHAT IS MICROSURGERY ANYWAY?

Two arteries about the same diameter as this "o" pass from the palm into each finger. The arteries become even smaller as they approach the fingertips, and they are proportionally smaller in children. The veins, which carry blood away from the fingers, are about the same diameter as the arteries, but they have a thickness and consistency similar to that of wet paper.

The survival of a finger is dependent upon these tiny blood vessels. But when an injured artery or vein is inadequately repaired, blood either leaks out of the vessel, clogs it, or both. In the past 30-40 years, surgeons have perfected specialized techniques and equipment to repair these digital blood vessels and similarly sized nerves. The adage that "what the eye can see, the hand can do" holds true for microsurgery.

It starts with a specialized, operating microscope where the surgeon and an assistant can sit opposite each other and view the same dime-sized area. The highly refined optics with magnification capabilities up to 40% of peak power require bright light, which has to be cabled from a distance to prevent heating of the illuminated tissues. Suspending this complex, heavy microscope over the operative field with the capacity to easily change its position and angle it, and then holding the microscope absolutely still, is no mean engineering feat in itself.

Delicate surgical instruments and steady hands come next. Nylon suture material almost invisible to the unaided eye secures the repaired blood vessels and nerves. The stainless steel needle fixed to the end of the suture is equally small and is sharp enough and thin enough to pass through a human hair.

It takes a microsurgeon about 15 minutes to place eight or nine sutures in a digital artery such that the blood flows through without clotting or leaking. We originally used these materials and techniques to reattach amputated fingers. Gradually these same techniques have expanded to allow the transfer of living blocks of tissue from one area of the body to another. For instance, to substitute for a missing thumb, we can detach the big toe from the foot and then attach it to the hand. The whole procedure may take up to 10 hours and usually requires a team of surgeons.

Various other deficits of bone, nerve, muscle, and skin, alone or in combination, are also correctable by microsurgical techniques. Microsurgery has greatly expanded the possibilities for restoring appearance and function in ways not thought possible in the recent past.

A GOOD ANIMAL BITE

During the first week after a microsurgical repair, the tiny, sutured blood vessels can clog. If the artery fails, the part turns white, and the only hope for salvage is another lengthy operation. If the vein fails, the part turns blue and swells up, just as if you had encircled your finger with a rubber band. Once the vein goes bad, the blood backs up and then the artery clots too. Can failed vein repairs be salvaged without further surgery?

Enter the medicinal leech. Replant surgeons keep a supply of these 2-inch blood lovers in the hospital pharmacist's refrigerator. The hungry leech attaches itself to the replanted part and draws off perhaps a teaspoonful of blood over 30-40 minutes. It then falls off in a stupor.

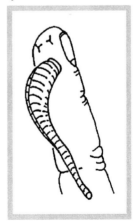

During its meal, it deposits a potent anticoagulant into the bite so that the wound continues to slowly ooze blood over the next 6-8 hours. This temporarily relieves venous congestion. The doctor or nurse then applies more leeches over the next few days until tiny veins have reconnected to permanently provide venous outflow.

Leech therapy is painless, and yes, repulsive. In the high-tech realm of replantation surgery, these low-tech animal bites have saved many reattached parts from failure.

Once the reestablishment of circulation is certain, the healing tissues and the concerned patient benefit from another specialist—the hand therapist.

WHAT EXACTLY IS HAND THERAPY?

We have a strong natural instinct to hold still when something hurts. But when a sore hand is held still too long, the injured tissues stick together and stiffness results. Conversely though, motion too soon or too energetic can increase the injury and delay recovery.

A hand therapist is a specially trained occupational therapist or physical therapist who maintains patients on the narrow path between too little and too much motion for the weeks or months required for optimal healing. The hand therapist helps the patient gently move joints without causing undue pain, strengthen necessary muscles, and gain confidence and skill in using the hand. Many therapists specializing in hands aspire to the CHT credential—Certified Hand Therapist, awarded after practicing hand therapy for a minimum of five years and passing a rigorous examination. The credential indicates a standard of excellence just as does board certification for doctors. You are likely to find a hand therapist near you by googling *Certified Hand Therapist* or *ASHT*. The therapist will need a prescription from your doctor before he or she can begin treating you.

Hand therapy methods include an initial warming of the hand, which softens the tissues and minimizes pain, followed by protected and progressive motion and strengthening routines. Because exercises must be repeated several times every day, the hand therapist's most important role is teaching the patient (and family, if necessary) an effective, safe home program.

Hand therapists are also adept at fashioning custom braces that may selectively immobilize and protect specific portions of the hand while allowing therapeutic motion to other parts. The plastic sheeting from which they mold these braces is fascinating. It softens readily in warm water, molds easily to the body, and then hardens to provide rigid support. Hand therapists are also great with gadgets and have a Pandora's box full of adaptive aids such as special spoons, high-tech scissors, button fasteners, and zipper hooks for individuals with restricted hand function. For every activity of daily living that the patient finds awkward or impossible, the hand therapist can usually show the patient an alternate way of doing it.

To coach apprehensive patients of all personality types and who are in pain through this rehabilitation process, hand therapists have excellent interpersonal skills and practice sidewalk psychology. They are all nice people—imagine holding hands at work all day. I say that hand therapists can make a patient cry and laugh at the same time. Some of the movements and activities the therapist requires of the patient border on uncomfortable, but the hand therapist charms the patient with distraction and encouragement so that he or she willingly returns for the next visit.

NONVIOLENCE ON TV

The wrist is a remarkable joint, or better put, a closely connected series of joints. Eight strangely shaped bones, each about the size of a sugar cube, are arranged snugly in two rows and link the hand to the forearm. When the wrist bones are working in concert, they allow for great flexibility and strength in positioning and using the hand.

So why would anybody want to watch the inside of a wrist on TV? The drama certainly can't compete with a soap opera, and you can find more action on *Larry King Live*. What "Wrist TV" lacks in entertainment, it more than makes up in value— particularly if you sprained your wrist six months ago and it still hurts. Here the "sprain" may actually be torn ligaments between two or more bones.

Ligaments are the tough, flexible connective tissues that hold bones close together. Small ligaments show up not at all on x-ray and poorly on magnetic resonance imaging (MRI). So having a look may be the only way to make a diagnosis. Until recently, having a look meant making a major incision that would open the wrist compartment enough to see the injury directly.

Unfortunately, this often causes additional damage and complicates the healing. Now, surgeons can view the interior of the wrist by making only a few ¼-inch incisions and inserting a lighted tube, which attaches to a small television camera.

Not only is the view of the wrist bones and their ligaments magnified and greatly improved, but also diagnosis and treatment can proceed with minimal additional injury. So here is one small instance wherein TV actually promotes nonviolence!

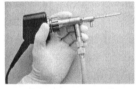

Endoscopy means "looking inside," and doctors have used lighted tubes to explore various internal body regions for generations. *Arthroscopy* is endoscopy of joints. The knee, because of its large size and vulnerability to injury, has been the prime site for arthroscopically assisted surgery over the past 30 years. Only in the last decade have arthroscopic equipment and techniques been miniaturized and perfected sufficiently to make wrist arthroscopy practical.

Now torn ligaments can be diagnosed and treated. Small bony fracture fragments can be teased accurately back into place, and severity of arthritis can be assessed precisely in order to focus treatment. Since the incisions required for arthroscopy are tiny, pain after surgery is minimized and patients go home the same day. They can immediately resume desk work and light manual activities such as channel surfing.

The finger joints are just too small for current arthroscopes to maneuver inside, and although elbows are large enough, the serious problems in the elbow call for more than what an arthroscope can deliver.

ELBOWS, OUR UNSUNG HEROES

Have you hugged your elbows today? You should. While hands and shoulders regularly receive praise for their function and grace, our elbows are quietly providing humble service. Elbows let us touch our feet and our ears. They also contribute to palm-up activities such as face washing and accepting change and for palm-down activities such as cutting food and using keyboards. Tendons strong enough to withstand body weight support this forgotten worker. These tendons permit straight-arm activities like cartwheels and bent-arm activities like chin-ups.

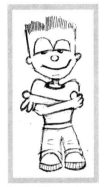

What can be done when elbows go bad, really bad, like when the joint is destroyed by rheumatoid arthritis, multiple fractures, a severe infection, or a tumor? Permanently stiffening the joint is not a good option since there is no compromise position that leaves the hand acceptably versatile.

In recent years, several interesting developments have occurred that allow for the reconstruction of a useful hinge between the shoulder and the hand. These high-tech innovations include replacement with metal and plastic, formation of scar in selective locations, or substitution with cadaver bone.

The development of a durable elbow implant has lagged behind the development of artificial hips and knees because the elbow has to withstand additional forces. We merely put pressure on our hips and knees, and we do that to our elbows too when pushing through a door. But we also put stretch on our elbows when carrying groceries and luggage. So a metal and plastic elbow replacement has to withstand forces that try to pull it out of the bone as well as forces that try to drive any total joint replacement farther into the bone.

After two decades of many false starts, total elbow replacement in the right patients has proven successful. The artificial elbow joint can restore a useful arc of painless motion for self-care activities, desk work, and light household activities. The implants can still pull loose, push loose, twist loose, become infected, and break. They will not withstand the forces necessary for playing tennis, hammering nails, or riding dirt bikes; there-fore, artificial elbow joints are reserved for older people with sedentary lifestyles. They work well in patients with rheumatoid arthritis who have multiple joints affected.

For a young person who has a bad elbow but has good bone and the ability to form good scar, using the patient's own tissues to reform a useful hinge is often the answer. Scar is good because it binds wounded tissues together. The challenge is to get scar to form solidly on the sides of the elbow to restore normal side-to-side stability and at the same time to prevent scar from forming on the front and back of the joint in order to maintain open-and-close mobility.

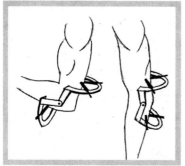

By placing the elbow in an elaborate contraption for about six weeks after a severe destabilizing injury, good stability and fair mobility can be restored. Steel pins drilled into the healthy bone above and below the elbow attach to an external frame. The frame is rigid from side to side. This rigidity protects the elbow from unwanted stresses while scar tissue has a chance to form and stabilize the joint. Furthermore, the frame is hinged and allows for elbow flexion and extension. Early and frequent elbow motion prevents dense scar from forming in areas that would normally stiffen the joint and prevent movement. The frame certainly looks strange, and the patient must be truly committed to wanting elbow motion back for the treatment to be successful, but it works.

The third means of restoring elbow function is especially useful when too much bone has been lost for either an artificial replacement or the scar modeling procedure to be considered. This entails replacing the missing segments of skeleton both above and below the elbow with the corresponding bone segments and supporting ligaments from a recently deceased donor. Temporary freezing of the graft eliminates rejection problems while maintaining the mechanical properties of the bone and ligaments. The graft is fixed to the patient's bones with strong steel plates and screws. Since supporting ligaments are included with the graft, the patient can begin moving the new elbow shortly after surgery. Over several years, the recipient gradually replaces the cadaver bone with his own. The joint surfaces, however, are never fully preserved. So once again, dirt biking, jackhammering, and cartwheeling are out.

The reconstructive possibilities for severely damaged elbows are innovative and useful. By no means do they restore normally functioning and durable joints. Have I convinced you that your own elbows are worth a hug?

What is possible when the forearm and hand are missing?

BIONIC HANDS

Artificial hands of one form or another have been around for hundreds of years. Originally they ranged from the extremely unsightly, intimidating, and somewhat useful (think Captain Hook) to reasonably aesthetic but entirely functionless (a gloved wood carving) attachments. Current versions have better function or appearance, but none excel at both. This may be changing. It comes as a consequence of war.

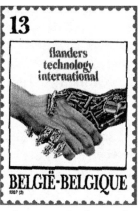

Sad as it seems, advances in surgery often result from the intense experience gained by treating war injuries. Fortunately, this experience then finds its way into civilian applications. Examples can be traced back nearly 500 years, to the time when surgeons learned that wounds healed better when they tied injured blood vessels closed rather than searing them with a red-hot poker. Less vivid and more recent advances include management of high-energy blast injuries and appropriate use of blood transfusions. The creation of hand surgery as a specialty was itself a product of war.

One good thing that stemmed from the conflict in Iraq has been a major advance in the form and function of artificial hands. Body armor saves lives, but these soldiers are too often left with hands and feet damaged beyond repair. The Department of Defense has initiated an advanced research project to address this large and largely unmet need. Understanding this engineering challenge says volumes about the complexity of the human hand and investigators' ingenuity to simulate it.

What is bionics anyway? Examples include studying dolphin skin to improve the design of boat hulls and understanding the way bats use echoes to enhance sonar and medical ultrasound. So bionics is the study of living systems for design application in nonliving systems.

The necessary features of a bionic hand start with the signal—how the user's thought to move the fingers turns into motion. Normally, this electrical impulse travels along nerves from the brain to the limb's muscles, which contract and move the joints. Presently when the wrist and finger muscles are missing, electrodes on the skin can pick up electrical activity in other muscles, which the user can learn to contract to signal the desired motion. This works but it is inefficient, similar to calling your neighbor and asking him to activate your garage door opener with his remote when you misplace yours.

In the future direct sensing from the ends of the amputated nerves or from the brain itself will offer far superior actuation. Of course the closer the sensor is to the nervous system's electrical activity, the more accurate the interpretation of the message will be. I doubt that many amputees would agree to have electrodes implanted directly on their brains with cords running out behind their ears, but most would probably opt for a hat or a headband with remote sensing capabilities.

Next comes mechanical power distribution. Over 40 muscles activate the wrist and hand normally. That many man-made motors strong enough to hold a tennis racket would be too big to fit inside an artificial limb. Smaller motors would be too weak to do the job. Fewer motors connected to cables running to the fingers may be a realistic compromise, but of course independent digital motions, such as for typing, are sacrificed. Under consideration are electric-motor alternatives that include inflatable balloons and metallic alloy strips that repeatedly change shape when heated or cooled.

Other issues include reducing the size and weight of the batteries and the computer needed to power and control the limb.

The prosthesis needs to be comfortable for prolonged use without causing skin irritation. The user should be able to squeeze firmly enough to open a jar and lightly enough to hold an egg and to know the difference.

The prosthetic's covering needs to be lifelike, tough, and easily cleaned. Inside parts need to be easily removed for repair or replacement. Components should be modular to take into account that one user's amputation is through the forearm and the next one's is through the upper arm. Then there are the issues of cost and durability. It is one thing to showcase the capabilities of an artificial hand in the lab where there are three engineers and a computer tech standing by. It is another thing to have these limbs in daily use on war veterans (thanks, again) and civilians as they go about their daily lives as normally as possible.

"AREN'T YOU GOING TO ORDER AN MRI, DOCTOR?"

I suppose 100 years ago when x-rays were in their infancy, patients were asking, "Aren't you going to order an x-ray, Doctor?" In the intervening century, doctors and patients understand pretty well when an x-ray could help make the diagnosis or plan treatment and when an x-ray would be superfluous. For instance, doesn't it seem appropriate that a sore tooth probably deserves an x-ray while a sore throat probably does not? In general, x-rays reveal structures that contain a high level of calcium--enough calcium to cast a shadow in the x-ray beam. Bones, teeth, hardened arteries, and kidney stones come to mind.

Doctors order x-rays with some caution, however, knowing that radiation in excess does bad things to bodies. Although that fact is well known today, it was not always so. For instance, dentists used to hold the film themselves when shooting x-rays of teeth. It was convenient and considered safe. Decades later the skin on their hands dried, cracked, and became cancerous. Now the person taking the x-ray steps out of the room before shooting the film, and there are well-accepted standards for how much radiation a person can receive on an annual and lifetime basis without undue risk.

We are now going through the same kind of learning curve with MRIs. Magnetic resonance imaging has been around for about 25 years. The machines are huge and hugely expensive. In essence, they are gigantic magnets, strong enough to make the subatomic particles in our water molecules wobble. When the magnet is turned on and off repeatedly, highly sensitive devices detect the faint electronic signal created by the wobbling protons. Computers then interpret these minute messages and create an image of the area being studied. In one common display mode, tissues that contain lots of water, fat for instance, show up as white. Tissues with less water in them, such as bone, are dark.

MRIs can identify problems in soft tissues that x-rays would pass right through without creating a shadow. MRIs are particularly useful when an organ without calcium, such as the brain or heart, is enclosed in a bony cabinet such as the skull or rib cage. MRIs can also be helpful in diagnosing problems in shoulders, hips, and knees, where large amounts of bone can shroud important soft tissue details from x-ray analysis. For several reasons, however, the same is not true for hands.

Compared to the heart or brain, the soft tissues of the hand are on the outside of the bone rather than inside, so they are accessible to the examiner's hand, never more than ¾ of an inch away. In a hip or knee, the problem spot could be three to four times farther away from the examiner's fingers and covered by several layers of fat and muscle. Also, a soft tissue injury in the hand can be big enough to hurt yet be too small to be accurately detected on MRI.

Hence, most hand surgeons have limited use for MRIs. There are times when they are helpful, but if you trust your hand surgeon, trust his or her judgment about when an MRI might be needed. One should be particularly wary of an attitude such as, "Well, I don't know what's wrong, so let's see if anything shows up on an MRI." A second opinion will definitely be cheaper and probably more valuable. Also, although current research shows that MRIs are safe, anything strong enough to make protons wobble makes me wonder. I just can't forget the dentist workers who unknowingly gave themselves cancer from those "innocent" x-ray beams.

AIRPORT SECURITY

Late for your plane, you hurriedly empty your pockets and rip off your watch. The TSA agent signals for you to proceed through the detector, the last hurdle between you and the boarding gate. Advancing bare-footed while holding your unbelted pants up with one hand and grasping your hard-earned boarding pass in the other, panic strikes. You remember that a

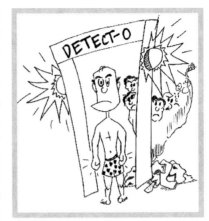

steel plate and screws support your recently broken wrist. Miss your plane? Strip search? Here is what really is going to happen.

The walk-through metal detector sends a pulsed magnetic field across the archway approximately 100 times a second. At the end of each pulse, the magnetic field reverses polarity and collapses at a speed recognized by the circuitry. A metal object passing through the archway retards the speed of the magnetic field's collapse. The alarm goes off. Maybe.

The size of the metallic object is important. For instance, dental fillings slip by, but sometimes so will a one pound hip implant. This is because the metal's composition has an effect. The plates, screws, and wires used for fracture fixation are traditionally made of stainless steel, which is about two-thirds iron. Some newer ones are made of titanium. Total joint replacements are often made from stainless steel or from an alloy of chrome, cobalt, and molybdenum. Each of these metals has its own magnetic signature, which means that some are more likely than others to set off the alarm. Then the detectors themselves have variable sensitivity; high, of course, when travelers are late. (Hint: Moseying or racing through the archway diminishes its detectability.) The wands are more sensitive than the archways, partly because the pulsing magnetic fields can be brought closer to your body and to any suspected metallic object.

Fat and muscle do not conceal implanted metal from the detector. Sorry. Also a note from your doctor is useless. Terrorists could forge one, so the TSA will ignore your doctor's note (probably illegible anyway) and use the wand and a through-clothes pat down.

The bottom line is this. If you have total knee and hip replacements, a spinal fusion, and plates and screws holding three fractures together, prepare yourself for the wand and a pat down. With less metal, it depends on the metallurgy and the mood of the machine. If the alarm goes off, the agent will screen you by hand and wish you bon voyage. Then be sure to fasten your belt before racing to the gate. Otherwise, you might get arrested.

HANDS IN SPACE

Travel into Earth's orbit has become almost routine as have space walks for repairing the Hubble telescope, inspecting the Shuttle, and assembling the international space station. What has been learned about hands since a Soviet cosmonaut took the first space walk in 1965?

First, the good news. Muscle strength and bone density in hands and arms do not deteriorate in space in contrast to hips and legs. Many returnees from space have been too weak to walk at first because their muscles atrophied from lack of use in the zero-gravity environment. Their arms and hands remained strong, however, because they were used to propel and stabilize themselves within the cabin and to control their tools and equipment both inside and out. This activity is sufficient to keep the hands and arms from getting flabby. Strengthening before the trip helps too because early space walkers noted hand fatigue from fighting the pressure and bulkiness of their gloves. This leads to the bad news.

The gloves are custom fit and quite complex. They withstand 600°F swings in temperature between sun and shade, fend off micro-meteors and protect the hand from the vacuum of space, yet permit dexterity. Usually the astronaut wears a thin fabric glove liner for comfort. The space glove itself is actually three gloves in one. The inner bladder is airtight with crinkles and ridges at the fingers and wrist to allow bending. The next layer, the restrainer, keeps the pressurized bladder in the shape of a hand rather than the shape of a balloon. The outer layer is the thermal micro-meteoroid shield. A heating system is controlled by a switch on the outside, which the space walker can flip on when working in the shade. The space suit itself but not the gloves also has a cooling system.

HAND SURGERY MEETS MOLECULAR BIOLOGY

When a mechanical part breaks or wears out, the correction is logically mechanical. These repairs, replacements, and substitutions range from the mundane (mending clothes, regluing furniture, changing tires) to the amazing (repairing the Space Shuttle in zero gravity).

Hand surgery, too, offers mechanical solutions for mechanical problems—realigning and securing fracture fragments, suturing injured nerves and tendons, replacing worn-out joints. Hand surgery though is more challenging than many other repairs because it deals with living people. Broken toasters, for instance, don't bleed, hurt, or feel compelled to play golf. That's the bad news for aspiring hand surgeons.

The good news is that hand surgery is easier in some ways than repairing a toaster, because once the living tissue is nudged back toward normal, the body can take over and complete the correction. Conversely a nearly repaired toaster cannot tighten its own screws.

Taking advantage of the body's capacity to heal is not unique to hand surgery, of course. If you have ever had sutures in your skin anywhere from head to toe, you know that the stitches go in, they come out, and then the skin continues to return toward its normal consistency, color, and feel over many months.

So surgical solutions for mechanical problems, right? Traditionally, yes, but wait. A narrowed artery is a mechanical problem, but many of these are now treated with blood thinners or cholesterol-lowering medications—chemicals! An amazing class is the body's own chemicals that signal resting cells to initiate repair of damaged tissues. Scientists are beginning to

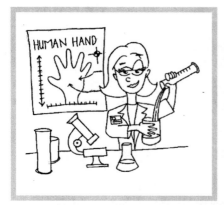

fabricate these messengers in test tubes, chick embryos, and even vats of bacteria. This blossoming field of molecular biology is vastly changing the entire discipline of medicine, even a specialty as mechanical as hand surgery. Here are three areas where musculoskeletal surgery is being replaced by molecular signaling.

Decades ago, Dr. Urist at UCLA discovered a protein extract that, when injected into the thigh muscles of mice, would induce the formation of bone at the injection site. It took years to identify the protein and then to determine its exact chemical structure. Of course, mice don't need hard calcium lumps in their quads, but surgeons use this protein to hasten bone healing after wrist fractures that would otherwise be problematic. The protein also serves as a bone graft substitute. Rather than supplementing the site of a spinal fusion with chips of the patient's bone to promote healing, surgeons can place cadaver bone laced with this bone-inducing protein at the fusion site. This saves operative time, diminishes the patient's discomfort after surgery, and accelerates recovery.

In rheumatoid arthritis, the body erroneously identifies its own cartilage as foreign and mounts an immunologic attack against this "invader." Damaged joints eventually destroy productive lives. Traditionally, doctors have used medicines such as steroids that blunt the body's immune response. These drugs protect the joints against the perceived danger, but they also diminish the immune system's response to actual dangers such as infections. Steroids also cause annoying side effects such as weight gain and easy bruising. This "shotgun" dampening of the immune system is now being replaced by highly focused medical treatments. For instance, researchers have identified the exact chemical messenger responsible for attacking cartilage and have concocted a protein that blocks its action. People still get rheumatoid arthritis, but with the early administration of this protein messenger joints remain healthy. Rheumatoid deformity, disability, and surgery are now avoidable.

Dupuytren's disease occurs mostly in men with northern European ancestry. Tight cords form in the palm and prevent the fingers from fully straightening. The problem becomes a daily curse during flat-hand activities such as clapping, shaking hands, face washing, and reaching into pockets. Dr. Dupuytren first described surgical removal of these benign but annoying cords in the 1830s, and the condition carries his name. In the intervening years, the treatment has remained surgical, which is generally helpful but necessitates a tender, swollen hand and an activity-limiting bandage for weeks. Under investigation is an enzyme that is injected directly into the cord and dissolves it. The enzyme shows promise for restoring full digital motion and becoming a quick and almost painless substitute for surgery.

Other, even more fantastic molecules are on the way. Of particular interest to hand surgeons are ones to enhance the quality and speed of tendon and nerve healing.

The next time you change a light bulb, which is providing a mechanical solution to a mechanical problem, think outside the box. "Could light bulbs be coaxed to repair themselves?" Certain cells can.

SOME NERVE!

My vote for the most amazing cell type in the body goes to the nerve cells that start in or near our spinal cords and run all the way to the tips of our digits. Other cells are so small that scores of them could hide under the dot at the end of this sentence. A peripheral nerve cell could wrap around this book several times, yet it is so fine in diameter that it would be invisible. Think about this. Your clock radio's electric cord has about 60 tiny strands of copper wire inside. Each of the two major nerves at your wrist is about the same diameter as an electric cord and has roughly 25,000 nerve fibers in it.

Consider, too, that nerves are capable of conducting electricity at 135 miles per hour, several times per second, for over 100 years. When a nerve gets cut, it does not die like other cells do--it tries to regrow to its original length!

The features that make nerves unique, however, also make them vulnerable to injury. When you cross your legs and your foot goes to sleep, it is because these cells are misbehaving for lack of oxygen. That effect may just be momentary. What about when a nerve is cut? If it is a "motor" nerve, the muscle it supplies is paralyzed. If it is a "sensory" nerve, not only is a patch of skin numb, you probably also will lose less-well-recognized capabilities.

For instance, reach your arm out and point your index finger away from you as far as you can. Now close your eyes and touch your index finger to your nose. Bingo. Or try this. Pinch three pages of this book with you left hand and only one page with your right hand. You can probably tell a difference in the thicknesses, which is only several thousandths of an inch. In each instance, specialized sensory nerves surrounding your joints tell your brain exactly how the joints are positioned so it knows precisely where your fingers are. As a result, you can find your nose in the dark or judge how far several sheets of paper are holding your thumb and index finger apart. Thank you, nerves.

So how do these amazing cells regrow? The control centers for hand and foot nerves, the cell bodies, are in or near the spinal cord. The only technical term you need to know is *axon*. This is the enormously long portion of the peripheral nerve cell that extends from the cell body to the muscle, joint capsule, or patch of skin for which the cell takes responsibility by conducting electrical messages. In groups of various sizes, the axons run in fibrous tubes, which insulate and protect them.

When an axon gets cut, the portion separated from the cell body degenerates, but the fibrous tubes remain intact. Within a week or so after injury, the cut axon begins to sprout finger-like buds, which seek the open tubes on the far side of the injury. In an incompletely understood and astounding manner, sensory axons tend to find their way back into fibrous tubes leading to the skin and joint capsules, and motor axons tend to find their way back into fibrous tubes leading to muscles. Molecular messengers stimulate the axon sprouts to find their way, and regrowth progresses about an inch a month. So if the cut is at the base of a finger, some sensation returns to the tip after about three months.

It gets a little more complicated, however, because when a nerve is cut the ends spring apart. If the ends of the fibrous tubes are not surgically reapproximated, the axon sprouts have trouble finding their way across the scar-filled gap, and they ball up in a confused mess.

If a nerve laceration is neglected for more than a few days or if a segment of the nerve is missing, then the gap needs to be spanned by a graft, which surgeons often take from the back of the leg. The fibrous tubes in the graft serve as conduits to guide the axon sprouts across the gap. Taking this leg nerve leaves a permanent numb patch on the foot, which is probably less irksome than a numb hand but not ideal. Also, the body has only a limited supply of expendable nerves that can be used for grafts. This becomes problematic when the gaps are multiple or lengthy.

Researchers have used sections of vein, strands of muscle, and cadaver nerves to coax regenerating axons across gaps. The best nerve graft substitutes may prove to be synthetic tubes. These keep the scar tissue out, which would thwart the axon sprouts' progress, and they are semi-porous so nutrients can pass through to nourish the axon sprouts. Then months later when the axons have spanned the gap, the tubes dissolve and leave no trace of their high-tech contribution to this regenerative phenomenon.

LIMB REGENERATION

Since nerves can regenerate, you may logically ask, "Why can't entire fingers, or even entire hands?" In some instances, they can—well, at least in salamanders. If one of these close relatives of frogs loses a leg, it grows back. If the salamander carelessly loses it again, no problem, it grows back. Some species of starfish have it even better. Not only can they regrow a missing arm, the arm can grow a missing starfish! The team trophy, however, goes to a particular worm, flat and about a quarter of an inch long. Cut one into as many pieces as you want, and each piece will generate a complete copy of the original. If this worked in humans, I can image basketball coaches wistfully eyeing their best players.

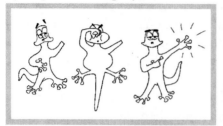

Scientists have studied salamanders extensively to understand this regenerative process. First, skin cells rapidly grow across the amputation stump and seal it. Then other cells, which in humans form scar tissue in this situation, migrate into the center of the injury zone. Here they clump together and change themselves into the same cluster of cells that formed the limb in the first place. This cell cluster grows into a replacement limb.

Think of it like this. A fire breaks out in the kitchen. The firemen arrive, isolate the fire to that area of the house, and douse it. For humans, they put up some plastic sheeting to protect what's left and leave. For salamanders, by contrast, the firemen huddle together in the debris, the captain says a few words, they shout "Yeah team!" and step apart. Momentarily, they all morph into infants, and then some turn into carpenters while others become plumbers, electricians, painters, or appliance experts. They pull out copies of the original blueprints and restore the kitchen to those exact specifications.

For living organisms, the blueprints are the genetic codes, which are contained in the DNA of each cell's nucleus. Pancreas cells read only certain portions of the code and produce insulin. Other cells read separate portions of the code and produce bone or gastric acid, for example. In most animals the ability to reread the blueprints and recreate the original design is lost after the original construction is complete. The code remains in place, however, and scientists are working on unlocking it.

The salamander studies reveal intriguing details. Make a scratch on a salamander's flank and it heals no differently than scratched human skin. Transfer a nerve ending into the scratched area, and the salamander makes a clump of cells identical to an embryonic limb bud, but it does not develop into a new limb. Add some grafted skin from other areas, and voilà, a limb forms right there on the animal's flank. It seems that the cell cluster uses chemical indicators from the wound, the nerve, and the skin grafts to get oriented, learn exactly what is missing, and then assign roles to various team members to produce muscle, bone, and all the other tissues necessary to reconstruct a limb.

Molecular biologists are identifying exactly which genes and which chemical messengers the wound, the nerve endings, and the skin activate and how they interact in this complex and amazing process. Some day, regeneration may offer the ultimate solution for injured or missing fingers or hands.

As fantastic as this seems, it is no more so than what we have already experienced—in 200 million years morphing from finny fish into Homo sapiens and in nine months growing from a single microscopic cell into a human being complete with tiny hands. These wonderful tools then grow, perform, and often repair themselves for a human lifetime, better when the owner provides proper maintenance. Human hands are beautiful in their compact complexity, capable of miraculous achievements, and worthy of our utmost respect. They are, nonetheless, just appendages. As miraculous as hands are, they are merely a reflection of the marvel of life in its entirety.

INDEX

A

Abbott, Jim, 69
acquired immunodeficiency
    syndrome, 121
Adams, Scott, 58
Agri, 11
Aizen My-o, 11
Akhenaten, 11
Allen, Rick, 70
American Sign Language, *54*, 59
American Society for Surgery of the
    Hand, *50*
American Society of Hand Therapists,
    188
amputation, 65
    digital, in surgeons, 65
    digital, ritualistic, *53*
    digital, story about, 66
    forearm, 121
Antwerp, Belgium, 175
applause, 166
arm pump, 81
arthritis, 121
    base of thumb, *33*
    rheumatoid, 121, 191
Assyria, 11
automobile, air bags, *45*
avocado, safe cutting, 108

B

Babylonia, 11, 13
bagel, safe cutting, 108
bank notes, 118
baseball
    curve ball physics, 79
    origin of southpaw, 75
Best Years of Our Lives, 71, 178
biology, molecular, 198
Bird-in-Hand, Pennsylvania, 126
blisters, 106

bone
    growth and maturation, 25
    growth and remodeling, 86
    physiology, 109
boxing, 86
braille, 56
Brandt, 152
Brandt, Mary Ann, 152
Britten, Benjamin, 70
bruise, 151
Buddhism, 12, 167
Buhl, Henry, 150
Bunnell, Sterling, MD, 142

C

calluses, 106
cancer
    fighting, 121
    nailbed, 133
carpal tunnel syndrome, *28*, 100
    endoscopic treatment, *30*
cartilage, *37*
casting materials, 6
Castle of Otrano, 176
Certified Hand Therapist, 188
Chief Left Hand, 74
chondroitin sulfate, *37*
Christianity, 12, 147
coins, 115
commandments, ten, 14
computer
    keyboard placement, *40*
    keyboard, modified, 71
    mouse, *40*
    use, *40*
cramp, writer's, 58

D

dance, gestures, 166
Daniele, Guido, 149